The Exercise Prescription
for
Depression and Anxiety

The Exercise Prescription
for
Depression and Anxiety

Keith W. Johnsgård, Ph.D.

Plenum Press • New York and London

Library of Congress Cataloging in Publication Data

Johnsgård, Keith W.
    The exercise prescription for depression and anxiety / Keith W. Johnsgård.
        p.   cm.
    Bibliography: p.
    Includes index.
    ISBN 0-306-43302-8
    1. Depression, Mental—Exercise therapy. 2. Anxiety—Exercise therapy. 3. Running—
Physiological aspects. I. Title.
RC537.J64   1989   89-15957
616.85′27062—dc20   CIP

For my children Paula, Mark, and Kris,
who persist in caring for me
despite my strange and mediocre ways

"Simply putting one foot in front of the other produces incredible results. It is no accident that the early California Indians called running, 'The Big Medicine.'"

—Len Wallach, Race Director,
Bay to Breakers

Preface

It has been my experience that educating men and women about lifestyle and its consequences can make a difference. Two years ago I organized a course at the university called "Exercise and Mental Health." With each semester the enrollment swells, and more and more students tell me that their experience in the course has significantly changed their lives. Some have stopped smoking or changed their eating habits, and many have given up their sedentary ways. Those who have begun regular exercise testify that it has elevated their moods, reduced their anxieties and tensions, helped them to deal with stress, helped them to lose unwanted pounds, and elevated their self-esteem. This book offers the reader much of what I share with students in that course.

Over the years I have become increasingly concerned with how we Americans have settled into the "Good Life," and the price that this new lifestyle exacts. Not so long ago we remained physically active throughout our lives, but we have now become a nation of sedentary observers. The great masses of us sit passively before our television sets or in stadiums and watch the talented few play games which used to be our own. The Centers for Disease Control tell us that our new sedentary lifestyle is the major health problem in America. It contributes importantly to the high rates of cardiovascular disease, osteoporosis, and obesity which trouble us. This book will suggest that we Americans have lost our way and are "unnaturally" depressed and anxious as a result of turning our backs on the active lifestyle which characterized all but our most recent past.

The Exercise Prescription is written for a variety of readers. Clinical psychologists and psychiatrists can use the book to inform themselves about the efficacy of exercise therapy for their patients. It compares exercise therapy to the current biochemical and psychotherapeutic treatments and includes case examples and suggestions for utilizing exercise as a primary or adjunctive treatment for depressed, phobic, and anxious patients. College students will find the book to be a single integrated source for information on exercise and mental health. But most readers will use the book to inform themselves about exercise and other mental health treatment options, and to intelligently prescribe exercise for their own depressions, anxieties, or stresses. The book is unusual in that it integrates information from a very wide variety of scientific fields. After becoming acquainted with the full spectrum of exercise's beneficent effects, the reader will be able to tailor a personal exercise program which can satisfy several individual concerns.

With such a diversity of potential readers, the book necessarily involves compromises. The professional reader and graduate student will find certain sections oversimplified, while some readers will find the same sections to be overly technical. The neurochemistry of mental disorders, for example, is far more complex than what I have presented, and, for that matter, far more complex than what we presently know. Some readers may skip over scattered technical sections which do not interest them. Other readers who desire even greater technical information than what is included in the text will find a large list of references which includes both significant recent investigations and important reviews.

While I wanted to write an understandable book about rather complex things, this is not a simple "how to" manual. You will find that it moves rather deliberately, developing important and necessary background information and concepts as it goes along. It therefore requires some patience, but when you reach the final chapter on the self-prescription of exercise you will be very well informed on a wide variety of exercise-related topics, and in a position to make intelligent and safe decisions about incorporating physical activity into your own life. The book should answer most of the questions you have about exercise and mental health.

If you're dismayed that so much of the book concerns running rather than other physical activities, I offer an explanation. Running is no better or worse than other aerobic activities, but because walk-jog programs are convenient, economical, safe, progressive, and easy to monitor, such programs have been the most widely used in research on exercise and mental health. Most relevant data concern running.

It's my hope that reading this book touches your life and causes you to to pause and consider how you are living. I have been physically active all of my life, but began distance running when I turned 50, and have run some 16,000 miles during the past decade. During that time I have belonged to running clubs, participated in countless races, and have run with men, women, and children in Europe, Africa, Asia, and across America. I have never met a depressed runner.

Keith W. Johnsgård

Monte Sereno, California

Acknowledgments

The first draft of this book took shape during a sabbatical leave when I lived at the Norwegian National Sports College (Norges Idrettshøgskole) in Oslo. Professor Gunnar Breivik was instrumental in bringing me there and helped make my stay intellectually stimulating and quite simply marvelous. The college provided me with free quarters overlooking the soccer field. It also provided a sports library, a typewriter, a ten-speed racing bike, an old Spanish guitar, a friendly cantina, a time of darkness, a time of unending daylight, and a lovely campus filled with men and women who were easy to know and love. It's a wonder I got any work done. But the Norwegian Marshall Fund had provided me with a research scholar grant to pay my travel and other expenses, so I worked as hard as I played. I am grateful to the Marshall Fund, the Idrettshøgskole, and the many Norwegian men, women, and children who opened their hearts and homes to me.

Running Times magazine and the Fifty-Plus Runner's Association provided subjects for my research concerning the motivation of long-distance runners, and I would like to thank the hundreds of men and women who took part in those studies.

Drs. Susan Backus, Peter Wood, and Ken Nishita supplied me with important reference materials. Peter, who is at the Stanford Center for the Study of Disease Prevention, and Ken, who is on the faculty at San Jose State University, also read sections of the manuscript. I am very grateful to these three professional colleagues.

Corky Smith typed the first draft of this book, and her frank emotional reactions to that early manuscript helped me keep the faith. When she began daily one-hour walks I believed that the book might have an understandable message of value. Thanks also to Dr. Frank Payne, my department chairman, who gave me an unrequested gift of time when I desperately needed it to meet the final manuscript deadline.

The shape of this book also reflects the many helpful criticisms and suggestions made by the consistently cheerful and supportive Plenum editors Linda Greenspan Regan and Victoria Cherney. This book is only somewhat related to the original manuscript which they received, but it is a better book. Freelance copyeditor Margaret Ritchie also helped teach me some things about writing and saved me considerable embarrassment. I owe all of these people, as well as production editor Andrea Martin, who put it all together.

Finally, I want to acknowledge the efforts of the hundreds of scientists and thousands of subjects who conducted and participated in the research projects which constitute the substance of this book. This is their story.

K.W.J.

Contents

Introduction

She didn't get to the part about the ice cream until we were well up the mountain. I had been silent since we had left our cars far below. An old hand at running mountains, I had learned long ago that it was a prudent thing to ask your partner a complex question when beginning a long uphill trail. Consequently I was running along real loose and breathing real easy. Debbie was struggling to consume enough oxygen to keep up with me and also tell me her story. When we left the car I had asked her how her day had been.

As days go, Debbie's had had a benign beginning. Her regular aerobics class and two hours of weight lifting at the gym had gone well during the morning. It was shortly after noon that things began to go down the toilet. She was scheduled to meet her husband Ted about then to go to an important funeral. One of his closest friends had died. But Debbie's mind was off on its own fast-moving journey as her body guided the family sedan down the freeway. She took a wrong exit and found herself in a totally foreign part of town. Immediately disoriented and already late, she panicked. After a terrifying trip against traffic on a one-way street she wound up sitting and sobbing at an intersection with honking traffic backed up behind her.

She missed the funeral and was overwhelmed with guilt. Familiar floodgates opened and her head began to swim in old and rancid self-depreciating waters. Wave after successive wave reminded her of what a scattered, undependable, and generally undeserving person she was. The beginning, it turned out, of a day that would become a world-class bummer.

We are moving through a cool, hushed, and shaded canyon of sweet-smelling bay trees when Debbie begins to tell me about the call. Lost and confused, she had double-parked and called Ted from a phone booth to report what had happened. He said he wasn't surprised, and was not able to wait for her any longer. He would go to the funeral without her. She related that he had sounded coolly indifferent. The worst sort of reaction, I thought silently.

Debbie must have thought the same thing because she left the phone booth, went straight home, and crawled into bed, funeral duds and all. On top of everything else, she would turn 40 the next day. She pulled the covers over her head, closed her eyes, pressed her hands over her ears, and curled up. Made sense to me.

By this time I am starting to feel pretty good. My muscles and joints are giving up the hope that I will turn around and point them back down to the car. They are warming to the task and grudgingly beginning to enjoy being useful. I hear them quietly opening a healthy discourse with the mountain, mumbling that they are going to win the battle on this particular day. By now they have recognized the trail and know that once we reach the top, a wondrous downhill awaits. They know that by then they will be in as good shape as they can hope for, and that during those last swift four miles downhill they can once again pretend that they are young. Meanwhile, I am thinking that it is good that Debbie got herself out of bed to run on this particular afternoon.

It's not an easy thing to find a good running partner, someone who is free to run at my favorite times, someone who likes the same distances, paces, terrains, and challenges—someone who shares my aversion to running before the sun is up. Debbie was all of those things and more.

In robust good health, she looked to be about 25, but she had been dealt a mixed genetic hand. While having to live with brain chemistry and mental processes which refused to ever slow down, she was blessed with an almost childlike face, wide-set eyes, nice high cheekbones, good skin, and a small frame she could work with. The years of running, aerobics, and obsessive, selective weight lifting had sculpted everything just right.

Running the trails with her was a little like watching an old Keystone Cops flick. Male runners who suddenly met us on the trail were invariably rendered senseless. Their eyes, obeying commands far older than themselves, would automatically lock onto Debbie. It was as if roller skates had been magically strapped onto their feet while they were suspended in the air in mid-stride. The consequences were something to behold. I would be running along behind, being super-cool, and smiling inside as I recalled how I had instantly lost awareness of my surroundings a month earlier when my eyes were reeled in by Debbie, who was standing in an adjacent checkout line.

In addition to getting my biweekly Keystone Cops fix, I was blessed with the added bonus of having long and tedious uphill sections brightened by Debbie's trusting and totally unfiltered stream of consciousness. Today's unraveling tale of disaster was the exception. I had never before seen Debbie depressed. In any case, her stories were never a burden. After earning a living by listening to troubled people for more than a quarter century, I had long since realized that there were only a few stories in life, but I was periodically awestruck by Debbie's style. She had a way of telling her story what was spellbinding. My runs with her lent weight to a growing suspicion that perhaps a real appreciation for style was as sensible and satisfying a goal in life as a quest for meaning.

Debbie's runs with me also offered her some bonuses. When I first met her she related that she had been searching for someone who would run hills with her in order to give her calves more "substance and definition." But a more significant bonus was a cost-free, half-dozen hours a week to run with a quiet shrink who was inclined to ask her how she was at the beginning of long uphill trails and then had the good sense to shut up—a listener who appreciated style.

It turned out that Debbie had spent several hours in the darkness under her bedcovers that afternoon. Eventually her daughter Allison returned home from a hard day in eighth grade. That got Debbie out of the bedroom. Still wearing her wrinkled black mourning outfit she stumbled out into a much more hazardous place. It was in the kitchen that her personal demon resided, and on this day increasingly dedicated to self-punishment, Debbie was a pushover.

Like an enamel Mona Lisa, the refrigerator sat patiently beaming as Allison began to hear her mother's confession. Mona knew that role reversals were a good sign, and it wasn't long before Debbie picked up on her inviting smile. This is the ice-cream part. Debbie started with sensible, but successive portions in a small dish, but the enamel lady soon convinced her that eating right out of the carton was just fine. Mona then suggested a second carton. Allison watched and listened.

With an OD history which was mostly limited to variations on a pasta theme, I had never in my life had any real interest in ice cream. This sudden twist in Debbie's story caught my attention. We had been running steadily uphill now for about 30 minutes and were not far from the top of the ridge. I figured I could safely break my vow of silence, so over my shoulder I inquired, "What flavor?"

When running in front of a partner on a narrow mountain trail, you have to guess what's going on behind, relying on whatever verbal cues you can pick up, but it was clear that my attempt at conversation caught Debbie's attention. Behind me, it turns out, she had been struggling to see through tinted contacts swimming in tears. She couldn't believe what she had heard. Stumbling on the trail edge she semishrieked, "What did you say?" Debbie frequently squealed but rarely shrieked.

Now the live oaks are thinning out and I am starting to catch breathtaking glimpses of the lake far below. I see a few long, slim racing sculls at their swift silent work. The trees are bunching up again, so without looking back, I repeat, "What flavor? You know, what flavor was the ice cream?"

A king-size surge of adrenaline catapults Debbie up beside me. While on a long odyssey in Nepal I had learned the hard way never to allow people and especially yaks to get between me and the uphill side of a narrow mountain trail. There, on the sometimes perpendicular roof of the world, it could mean the difference between life or death. It was now automatic. So Debbie is stumbling along the crumbling edge of this nasty trail section, leaning forward and looking into my face demanding eye contact. Except for the very briefest moments, I always keep my eyes on the trail when moving—another Himalayan lesson. This further incenses Debbie.

"I can't believe that I heard what I just heard," says Debbie with feeling. She talks that way. She goes on, "You call yourself a psychologist and you want to know the flavor?" She casts her eyes to the heavens, now into serious shrieking, "He wants to know the fucking flavor!"

We run a silent 100 yards and I hear Debbie say quietly, and mostly to herself, "I hate myself when I eat."

Another 100 yards unravel and she speaks a little more loudly, chiding me, "You ought to know that."

Silence once again; then I hear her mutter, "And he calls himself a shrink."

I'm running along thinking that I am glad that I'm her running buddy and not her shrink. I am segueing into being grateful that her problems are hers, and not mine, when we pass through a beautiful stand of tall madrone trees. Their peeled, orange trunks and branches are chalky-dull, but their big, deep green, ovate leaves shine softly in the late afternoon sunlight. My thoughts flash back to the previous November, and how I had unexpectedly burst into tears when I first saw those same deep green leaves on rhododendron trees after weeks in the rarified air and sterile world of ice and rocks high above the clouds in Nepal's Solo-Khumbu. Debbie brings me back to California.

"It's bad enough to be ding-y," she says quietly.

We are moving out of the madrone grove 50 yards later when she finishes with, "I can't stand being both fat and ding-y."

I register that silently. I'm once again beginning to catch staccato glimpses of the lake shimmering below. The rowers, now motionless, are coasting along, their raised and dripping paddles backlighted by the brilliant late afternoon sun.

Debbie, whose anger has crested, has tucked in behind me and the lake disappears, so I decide to give it another try. "Yeah," I throw back over my shoulder, "I was curious about the flavor."

We work our way around the edge of an open grassy knoll. A meadowlark breaks cover beside the trail and tries to lead us away from her nest. Her song sends me back to my childhood on the prairie. Then I wonder why she chose to build her nest so close to the trail, what with all that open wild space. I am beginning to sink into the sterile quicksand of philosophical metaphors when Debbie rescues me.

I hear her softly murmur, "Steve's Cookie Monster."

I let that sink in for more than 50 yards, all the way up into the sudden deep shade of the live oaks. It's hard to coax heavy stuff into the left brain when running up a mountain.

Then I ask, "Both cartons?"

A substantial silence ensues; then comes the delicious, fantasy-provoking answer.

"French Vanilla with Crushed Chocolate Bits and Cherries."

I can almost taste it, but behind me it sounds as if Debbie is having trouble breathing. I figure that her emotions must be re-shaping back there. We are momentarily backed up against the mountainside as a pair of mountain bikers career down past us. We scarcely break stride, and once they are past and we have settled back into a steady pace, I toss back, "I've never heard of Steve's Cookie Monster. How is it?"

"Really good!" gasps Debbie, who is now breaking up with laughter and falling behind.

It was a memorable run. The last four miles would have been spoiled by talk. We came down the mountain on a fresh spring wind, flowing through the river gorge and down into the valley at a swift pace which neither of us would have sustained alone. A couple of times I thought that we were a pair of coyotes.

When we reached our cars at Forbe's Mill, Debbie's obsessive, self-punitive thoughts and her depressed mood seemed to be completely gone. She was heading home in a much improved mental state, one which would keep her out of bed, out of the refrigerator, and out of a potentially explosive spousal scenario.

So what do we have here? Is this an example of how running therapy reduced an acute depressive episode and drove a definitive wedge into obsessive rumination? Maybe. Maybe not. Debbie's mountain run raises a number of questions. There are all sorts of possibilities as to what happened on the mountain that summer afternoon.

Did Debbie feel better because she was able to tell me her story and expiate her guilt as we ran up the mountain? And if it was the confession that was critical in helping her to feel better and better about herself, was I necessary? Could she have just as well told her story to the mountain, or could she just as well have told it to any running partner who was a good listener but didn't carry a clinical psychologist's credentials?

But Debbie's story was more than just a simple confession. It was a powerful and explosive cathartic experience. The anger which she had turned inward on herself during the preceding hours burst out and was directed at me. Would that outburst have occurred with another running friend who would have perhaps been talking sympathetically and been overly supportive all the way up the mountain? Debbie might have instead responded to the supportive friend with a whole series of "Yes, buts" to justify why she should persist in despising herself.

Another possibility is that there were some psychologically relevant physiological changes produced by the run. It could be that her high inner body temperature gave rise to a wonderfully tranquil state, a condition which could have been attained with considerably less effort through a visit to the sauna. It's also possible that the running resulted in significantly increased activity by various antidepressant or euphoria-producing neurotransmitters in the pathways and areas of her brain which regulate mood.

Another possibility is that the change in Debbie's mood was the result of cognitive processes which interacted with the emotional and other physiological processes. Cognitive processes include a variety of higher mental processes such as thought, perception, memory, and awareness. One possibility is that the stressful run might have distracted her and broken up a self-perpetuating ruminative system of increasingly depressing thoughts about what a terrible person she was. Perhaps the right movie could have distracted her just as well.

Humor could also have played an important cognitive role. After silently listening to her tragic story for the course of a full half hour, my first question was about the flavor of the ice cream. It immediately infuriated her, but when I later spoke for the second time inquiring about the flavor of the second carton she began to break up with laughter. Some sort of cognitive-emotional interaction took place which allowed her to reframe the whole episode and make it less tragic. While it remained a serious experience, it was neither unforgivable nor the end of the world. My behavior that day was not entirely unpremeditated and thoughtless.

There are other processes which could have been involved. Perhaps, for example, it is very difficult or even impossible to run strenuously and to be depressed at the same time. These two physiological states may well be antagonistic. If that is so, there are a couple of ways that cognition might be involved in the process. The first is that how we humans feel at a given moment may have something to do with what we think about or what we remember. Maybe we are less likely to think about depressing things during the highly energized state of running. Another possibility is that if Debbie has learned that running always provides dramatic relief from acute depressive episodes, she possesses a very powerful tool to care for herself. She has the capacity to effectively deal with her moods—a cognitive awareness of self-mastery and an internal sense of control.

There may be other possibilities, but a more basic question remains. Did the run actually reduce Debbie's acute depressive mood, or did it simply produce feelings of well-being? Since the level of her depression was not assessed objectively either before or after she ran, this question is unanswered.

An even more serious issue is the possibility that the symptom relief which Debbie experienced after the run actually did her a disservice by decreasing the likelihood that she would seek out needed professional help. If Debbie actually suffered from some sort of mental disorder, running could be viewed as a psychological crutch which allowed Debbie to perpetuate her psychopathological ways.

If Debbie suffered from a chronic depression, her exercise must have constantly ameliorated its symptoms, for she never acted depressed nor did she ever complain to me about feeling depressed. Debbie presented a mixed picture. She was very externally oriented, depending on other people, particularly men, to affirm her as a person. She was quite dependent, obsessive about her appearance, compulsive about her body, and completely unconscious of her seductive manner of dressing and behaving. Together with her daily workouts these symptomatic behaviors could well have covered and eased a chronic depression. Debbie didn't feel very good about herself and she was convinced that her marriage was without hope.

But Debbie was much more than what her attention-getting persona would suggest. I came to experience her as a warm, empathic, honest, and caring woman. She was marvelously open with regard to whatever was consciously available to her, perhaps trusted others too much, and had a sense of humor that was a gift to those around her. She would often do and say things which would unexpectedly cause me to laugh out loud. Real belly laughs. I just appreciated who she was.

If you have invested thousands of dollars and countless hours in psychotherapy, you are likely to view Debbie's running therapy with considerable skepticism. It makes sense that you would see her run as no big deal—only superficial symptom reduction and temporary respite from deep-seated and unresolved emotional problems which will surface again and again until Debbie does as you have done and arrives at your level of awareness and self-acceptance. Maybe.

But even on the day of our run, Debbie had some things which you may still be without. She possessed some guaranteed and cost-effective personal skills which allowed her to quickly break out of periodic acute depressive episodes. These skills also allowed her to interdict occasional periods of uncontrolled self-depreciating rumination before they became disabling and dangerous. Finally, she was supremely healthy, had almost no body fat, and looked smashing. Nobody's perfect.

As time went on I would discover that Debbie had spent considerable time in psychotherapeutic treatment. Alone, or with her husband, she had seen three different therapists over the course of several years. Her therapeutic experiences had ranged from moderately helpful, through benign, and on to destructive. She had finally given up on psychotherapy and had settled for being the same old Debbie with the same old demons. She figured that when push came to shove, it always came down to her own decisions and her own resources. She took care of herself as best she could.

When autumn came along the shorter days reminded me that I would soon have to return to the university, and that my runs with Debbie would become infrequent or would even end. Before that happened I had a long talk with her. I told her that I had talked with a special, trusted colleague about her, and that she had agreed to treat Debbie if she wished. I explained that my friend was a first-rate therapist and that she specialized in working with women who had problems similar to Debbie's. I mentioned that she worked in a public agency which charged according to a sliding fee scale, and I pointed out how that would make it possible for

Debbie to see her for as long as was necessary, regardless of which direction her life might take. That was a couple years ago, and Debbie is still in treatment.

It is precisely because Debbie's run asks more questions than it answers that it serves to lead into the longer and more complex story which follows.

In order to answer the questions which Debbie's story raises, it's important to know just what sorts of mental problems most commonly trouble American men and women. Is depression common enough to warrant our attention, and are there different kinds of depression? It's also important to consider the causes of depression and anxiety, and to take a special look at their biochemical aspects, since psychoactive drugs, coping styles, stress, and exercise can all impact the biochemical systems which affect our moods.

Then there is the question of treatment and efficacy. Just exactly how effective are the current biochemical and psychotherapeutic treatments when it comes to dealing with the symptoms of depression and anxiety? Are they better than nothing? If so, just how much better? We need a standard against which to judge and compare the effectiveness of exercise therapy.

And finally, since lifestyle importantly affects our internal chemistry and moods, it is important to begin by recalling how we humans lived before the time of tranquilizers, antidepressant drugs, psychotherapists, and cookie monsters.

Chapter 1
The Violation of Our Genetic Warranty

We human beings are very recent. It has been commonly accepted that early Americans and their wolf dogs came down from Alaska about 12,000 years ago, flooding out of the glacier-free Yukon Corridor and spreading across a great game reserve that would one day be called the United States. But there is recent evidence which suggests that earlier pathfinders may have found their way across the Bering Land Bridge and down onto our great plains 26,000 years ago and may have painted Brazilian cave walls as long as 32,000 years ago. However, it was about 10,000 years ago that our ancesters fully occupied and laid claim to what is now the United States. At about that time some were building huge stone pictographs on the surface of the southwestern deserts, pleas to the water gods to stop the drying of the earth and the disappearance of the woolly mammoths, mastodons, giant camels, and giant bison.

Some 5000 years ago, about the time the pyramids were going up in Egypt, some of us had settled into the floodplains of eastern rivers and began to farm. We raised squash, sunflowers, and other domesticated native plants. Eventually we moved up into the adjacent hills and ridges, clearing away the forests of native oak and hardwoods. More than a thousand years before Columbus "discovered" America we had begun to cultivate corn along the Little Tennessee River. Some of the virgin forests which Daniel Boone explored were second-growth evergreens and cedar, and some of the "savages" he met were longtime farmers.

We early Americans were *Homo sapiens sapiens,* "man the wise," Cro-Magnon man, the selected survivors of a long series of evolutionary experiments which had begun nearly four million years earlier when our distant ancestors first began leaving footprints across central Africa. We were children of the last ice age. Our prototypes took shape about the same time as the great glacial ice masses began to form some 70,000 years ago. About 35,000 years ago our distant cousins, the Neanderthals, abruptly vanished, leaving us alone, the last of the line. Those of us who, by torchlight, used sticks to paint bison on the cave walls of France were the same as those of us who now spraypaint graffiti on the walls of New York subways. Our customs and language have changed, but we are the same.

Our time is brief, a passing squall in the immense evolutionary rainstorm which has spawned life on this planet for hundreds of millions of years. But we have a clear genetic legacy, and it is becoming increasingly apparent that if we stray too far from the lifestyle which we lived when we were so carefully selected, we put ourselves at serious risk.

In pursuit of consciousness and civilized ways we have left much of ourselves behind, disrespected and disowned. We have relinquished our spiritual bonds with, and our respect for, the plants and animals with whom we must cooperate and coexist if life is to go on. We have stopped listening to the voices which sing within our souls, and we have stopped respecting and attending to our dreams. Prisoners of distressingly narrow and irrelevant skills in an increasingly complex world, we are less and less able to do for ourselves.

And we have become sedentary. The original High Plains Drifters, we had foraged and hunted across the sky-swept savannahs, the pursued and the pursuers, forever on our feet, and always on the move. With spear in hand we flowed with the passing millennia on a seemingly endless journey into the slow dawn of civilization.

As little as 10,000 years ago we all still lived as hunter-gatherers. By 2000 years ago about half of us had stepped from our ancient path to become farmers and herders. As time went on our ways became increasingly divergent from how we had lived when we were so carefully selected as the sole survivors of that long line of man-apes.

But even as recently as a century ago here in America, most of our lives involved long hours of hard physical labor and a diet reasonably similar to that of our forebears. The lifestyle of the late 1800s still fell within the design specifications of *Homo sapiens sapiens*. Our Cro-Magnon physiological systems with their interdependent functions and feedback mechanisms still worked. But the 1900s brought previously undreamed-of lifestyle changes, and the consequences were both wondrous and disastrous.

Life Expectancy Soars

Average life expectancy 2000 years ago, at the time of Christ, was only about 25 years. Not much time to get it all done. When Lincoln was addressing the folks at Gettysburg, the kids who were playing cowboys and Indians out beyond the crowd weren't all that much better off. Their average life expectancy was only about 40 years—up only 15 years over the course of two millennia.

But today's babies can expect to live an average of an astounding 75 years. If you recently became a parent you may be thinking that they ought to come with a longer warranty, since they cost so very much. But what we have here is something truly remarkable. After all of these thousands of years, in little more than a single century life expectancy here in America has nearly doubled.

Life, however, still has a limit. Our maximum life potential (MLP) was set about 50,000 years ago when we first came off the drawing board. The Hayflick Limit[5] (the maximum number of times our body's somatic cells will divide before obeying an ancient genetic order to call it quits) differs for each animal species. For example, the limit is 28 doublings for mice, which have an MLP of four years. The huge Galapagos sea turtles are allowed a maximum of 125 doublings and 175 years. We average about 50 doublings. Our limit is 60 doublings and we have a 115-year maximum life potential.

So what's all the fuss about? We are living twice as long as we did only about a century ago, and we are getting closer and closer to our genetic limit. There is considerable to fuss about. For starters, we aren't all average. We are each dealt a unique genetic hand which can range from virtually bullet-proof to dreadful. Once born, we play our hands differently. Some of us live in ways that maximize our genetic potential while others knowingly or unknowingly invite early death. And sometimes, of course, we are forced into games we don't choose. Even with a good hand and a thoughtful and cautious life, we can get suddenly erased—as by a drunk driver. Cultural and socioeconomic factors figure heavily in the habits and lifestyles which impact our life expectancies. Not all of today's babies will live the average 75 years, and many will invite long years of disability and pain before prematurely dying.

Other things being equal, for example, today's white girl babies can expect an extra 4 years. Black boy babies can expect 10 fewer. Babies who become lifelong alcoholics can subtract a dozen years. Smokers, who will die prematurely from a host of tobacco-related diseases, will lose 5 to 9 years (depending on how much they smoke) and will be often be incapacited by heart and lung disease or cancer for several additional years before dying. Years can be subtracted increasingly as obesity swells. In addition to eating too much, today's babies can also eat away precious years by adopting unnatural diets, eating far too much saturated animal fat and avoiding the unprocessed complex carbohydrates for which our digestive systems were designed. Finally, babies who become couch potatoes will die prematurely, and those who remain active throughout their lives will live longer.

The Good Life

We Americans seemed intent on killing ourselves. Around mid-century we settled into a kind of suicidal, immediate- gratification binge. We sat around stuffing too much of the wrong sorts of things into our mouths—trading immediate relief for potential addiction, future disability, and premature death.

We gave our children to television and our games to professionals. We no longer had to provide our own mediocre heroics or, for that matter, even participate, in order to enjoy sports. Our dollars were funneled into making the very talented few better. We built great arenas and stadiums. We bought recliners and TV sets. We became a nation of increasingly non-heroic overweight observers.

Those were the years of the Good Life. The big war was over and we had won, emerging as a world power. Most of us who wanted to work had jobs, and families could get along fine with only Dad working. Veterans could buy decent houses for $5,000 with nothing down and a 3.25 percent loan. The GI bill made college possible for people who never dreamed of higher education. After years of rationing, hard times, and doing without, we could now afford two cars in every garage, at least one TV, T-bones on the barbecue, season tickets for the ball games, incredible food selection the year around, all the cigarettes we could smoke, and all the booze we could drink. Labor-saving home appliances and power equipment made sweating something we did only beside the pool.

While we may have looked like a herd of contented cows licking our way around the Big Rock Candy Mountain, our bodies were in crisis. Designed to run on physical activity and 50,000-year-old menus, we asked them to adapt to substances which weren't around during our evolution. We coughed, vomited, spit up blood, staggered, and sometimes became unconscious. And those were only the acute initial reactions to some of the 20th-century substances we asked our bodies to get used to. The bad stuff, the lethal chronic effects, came later.

It's not hard to understand why we all dipped so deeply into the Good Life punch bowl. It was marvelously seductive, and the bleak effects of the habits which would disable and prematurely kill us were insidious and unhurried. The slow but steady increases in blood pressure and heart rate whispered only softly of arteries which were slowly plugging. We didn't notice. We forgot that there were now-distant mornings when we awoke without coughing and times we climbed stairs without being left breathless. We were always surprised when we felt those first sharp and unfamiliar chest pains which signaled a cardiac event. We couldn't believe the chest X rays which spoke of cancer and told us that the odds were only 1 in 10 that we would live another five years.

The habits which will plug our arteries, scar our livers, and turn our lungs into uneasy radioactive tar pits are laid down in youth, a time when we most strongly feel the urge to follow the crowd and mimic adults, a time when we just can't wait for time to pass so that we can get on with things. As kids, it seems we will live forever. Perhaps we carry this myth with us into adulthood, the myth that we are somehow special, and that the odds and rules which apply to other people don't have much to do with us. Perhaps that is why we go right on doing the things which will kill other people.

A Change in the Nature of What Was Killing Us

Medical historians are going to look back and marvel at the 20th century. Besides the near doubling of life expectancy, there was this curious twist in the nature of what killed us. When the century began, we were victims of other killers, but 50 years later we were busy killing ourselves.

In 1900 almost all of us died of infectious acute diseases. Tuberculosis accounted for an astounding two-thirds of our deaths. Today hardly anyone dies of TB, smallpox, typhoid, diphtheria, and all of those early killers. Only influenza and pneumonia remain uncontrolled, and deaths from these illnesses occur almost without exception among the very old or people who are already seriously ill.

It is of significance that the sparing of millions of lives and the dramatic increase in average life expectancy during this century are almost completely the result of improvements in hygiene, diet, and preventive medical care. They reflect the consequences of *prevention* rather than advances in biomedical knowledge regarding treatment of the infectious diseases which used to kill most of us.

Today nearly all of us will die from chronic diseases. Cardiovascular diseases such as heart attacks and strokes will kill half of us, cancer will kill a fourth, and things like cirrhosis, emphysema, and diabetes will take up a large part of the remaining slack.

You are probably figuring that this makes sense—that with acute diseases licked, we now live long enough to develop the chronic diseases which come with aging. There is some truth to that line of thought. But epidemiologists Drs. Jim Fries and Lawrence Crapo[4] of the Stanford University Center for the Study of Disease Prevention point out that chronic diseases are not simply the *natural consequence of aging*. They appear, in large part, to be the consequence of an *unnatural lifestyle*. A poor genetic hand will predispose some of us to cardiovascular (CV) disease, for example, but as many as half of us who develop such disorders will do so because of how we live.

Culture and Disease

Consider the fact the CV disease is unknown in about three fourths of the world. Again, you may be thinking that this is because people in more undeveloped areas don't live long enough to plug up their arteries. Perhaps, but there are some small and remote contemporary communities which contain unusually high percentages of healthy and active people between the ages of 80 and 100, people free of CV disease. Scientist Alexander Leaf [7] studied three isolated villages high in the Andes Mountains of South America, the Karakoram Mountains of Pakistan, and the Caucasus Mountains of Russia. The people in these remote villages have not stepped far off the lifestyle path of our ancestors, and although they are separated from one another by great distances, their lifestyles reflect a number of common denominators. Diets are low in both calories and animal fat, tobacco and alcohol are used in moderation, and no one ever retires. Men and women remain physically active, enjoying unusually high levels of fitness throughout life. Only death cancels the purpose and meaning in the lives of these people, who never cease working in the fields or participating in village affairs.

How we live has a great deal to do with how long we will live, and with what will kill us. The Japanese, whose low-fat diets include prodigious amounts of salt and smoked fish, suffer from diseases somewhat different than those which afflict us here in high-saturated-fat America. But if Japanese immigrate to this country and pick up our habits, the nature of what kills them begins to change. They trade hypertension and stomach cancer for cardiovascular disease.

A few years ago Dr. Lester Breslow, dean of the UCLA School of Public Health, pointed out that destructive forms of behavior have put the United States near the bottom with regard to health when contrasted with other nations in the Western world, even though we spend more of our national resources for health than any other country. Keynoting the fourth National Conference on High Blood Pressure in Los Angeles, Dr. Breslow cited "antilife habits" as responsible for the fact that an American man of 40 has less chance of living to be 50 than his counterparts in almost all of the industrialized European nations.

Consider what would happen if we Americans made only three important lifestyle changes. If we stopped smoking, drank in moderation, and controlled our blood pressure, we would cut our hospital admissions in half according a University of Tennessee study reported by that school's Center for Health Sciences. In America more than 1 out of every 10 dollars of our gross national product goes to health care.[3] If we suddenly began to live sensible preventive lifestyles it would precipitate a national crisis. Pharmaceutical companies, hospital suppliers, doctors, nurses, health insurance companies, hospitals, and all of the related support people and purveyors would be affected. Millions of people would be out of work. In a sense, our current economy depends on our making ourselves mortally ill. Of the deaths due to chronic disease in America, the Centers for Disease Control estimate that as many as 50 percent can be traced to lifestyles which violate our genetic warranty.

Organ Reserve

While the Hayflick Limit is genetically fixed, a second important factor which affects our life span, organ reserve, is highly plastic. Most of us possess far more organ reserve than we require to simply get along. We can, for example, function quite well with only partial kidneys or livers, or with only a single lung. Our heart rate can be increased many times over its resting rate when conditions demand—handy when chasing woolly mammoths or being chased by saber-toothed tigers. This reserve capacity allows us also to maintain life-critical internal balances when we are stressed by trauma or illness. Fortunately, kids are born with incredible reserves and can survive major traumas that would quickly kill very old people.

Organ reserve gradually diminishes with age. For example, our maximal allowable (safe) heart rate is figured at 220 minus our age in years. Thus, what is playful exertion in youth can be life-threatening in old age. But organ reserve responds dramatically to how we live. We can diminish it and in some cases increase it.

Smoking, for example, alters our blood chemistry and contributes to the plugging of our arteries. These processes, together with smoking's other chronic effects on our lungs, seriously reduce our cardiorespiratory reserve. The carbon monoxide in cigarette smoke reduces oxygen in our blood and can produce cardiac arrhythmias (heartbeat irregularities). Blend these chronic and acute effects of smoking with stress, and you have trouble in River City. Those of us who suffer sudden death while playing golf are often heavy smokers. Some of us who are sedentary heavy smokers may not possess the cardiorespiratory reserve for mowing the lawn without risk.

Those of us who drink heavily will progressively scar our livers, eventually leaving ourselves just enough functional liver tissue to get along, provided that we don't run into serious trauma or injury. A case of hepatitis, which would involve moderate risk for a light drinker, would be a death notice for those of us who have drunk away our liver reserve.

Use It or Lose It

But there is good news. Many of the physiological systems which are so critical to our well-being are remarkably plastic, adjusting nicely to what we ask of them. Muscles, for example, not only get larger and smaller with use or disuse but also react to the specific kinds of demands we make on them. Bones, too, are plastic. If you want bird bones, perch. If you want gorilla bones, forage.

The best of all possible news is that while CV disease is our biggest national health problem, our CV system is perhaps the most plastic of our systems. We can ruin it by putting the wrong sorts of things in our mouths, but we can also swell its reserve capacity with use. In fact, the emerging view of many chronic diseases such as coronary heart disease and osteoporosis (porous bones which crumble and easily break) is that they are *diseases of disuse* rather than the consequence of overuse associated with accumulating years. Taking it easy can be poor advice indeed.

Fries and Crapo[4] remind us that while cardiorespiratory reserve does slowly decrease with age, it is far more variable within a given age group than between age groups. For example, a well-conditioned 50-year-old man isn't all that different from a well-conditioned 20-year-old man. However, he is very different from other 50-year-olds. Consider the marathon, an athletic event on which we possess considerable statistics. An overweight and sedentary 50-year-old man who is a heavy smoker, if forced to participate, would very likely collapse and could even die near the starting line. Other healthy, but normally sedentary 50-year-old men could require two or three days to complete the 26.2 mile race. However, a well-conditioned 50-year-old man who finishes with an average time of about 3½ hours would possess cardiorespiratory fitness greater than nearly *all men of all ages*. But to be the fastest 50-year-old, he would have to reduce his finishing time by about an hour. A fast 70-year-old man could finish in under 3½ hours. If our well-conditioned marathoner stops exercising regularly, his cardiorespiratory fitness would adjust to the demands of a sedentary life and would rapidly drop off to a level which would provide only minimal reserve in case of serious trouble.

If it seems remarkable to you that an ordinary 50-year-old might, through training, develop the cardiorespiratory fitness of someone 20 to 30 years younger, consider the following. At the 1987 World Veterans' Track and Field Championships in Melbourne, Ed Benham, an 80-year-old from Maryland, ran the 10,000 meters (6.2 miles) in slightly over 45 minutes, and 94-year old Jing-Chang of Thailand ran a 48-second 200 meters (slightly more than one lap around a standard American quarter-mile track). Azad Singh Phithvi of India, who was 97, competed in the 100- and 200-meter events. Older runners consider 50-year-olds to be youngsters. America is graying, but aging is being dramatically redefined.

Prevention versus Repair

It is important to bear in mind that the two major causes of death in America, heart disease and cancer, are unlikely ever to be "cured" by advances in biomedical research. It would be imprudent to count on it, at least in the near future. For the most part, our current technologies can only decelerate the progression toward early death. Paradoxically about 93 percent of the money spent on health care in America is spent on medical care for the sick.[6] The key to dealing with our two primary killers is prevention, but we spend only a tiny fraction of our health dollars on research, education, and programs to help us turn our backs on our newly acquired antilife habits. We have lost our way and we are paying the price.

If our nation's primary health problem is largely self-imposed chronic illness, the role of medicine should be focused as strongly on prevention as on repair. Prudent consumers should be able to seek out physicians who, within the boundaries of responsible judgment, encourage them to live a preventive lifestyle, bearing in mind that exercise is an increasingly common prescription for even the most serious sorts of health problems. It is even wiser to seek out physicians who themselves exercise. They are going to be around longer and are better able to understand the common problems which trouble active people who have chosen periodic muscle and tendon pain over terminal chest pain. Such physicians would also be inclined to cast an irreverent eye on our contemporary notions of normality. Later in this book we will see that experts question our current standards for things such as ideal body weight and acceptable blood cholesterol levels. For example, "normal" resting pulse rate and blood pressure in America might be substantially different if we all lived the species-normal lifestyle which characterized our ways not so very long ago.

Twentieth-Century Depression

There is ample evidence that our physical health has been significantly impacted by our radically new lifestyle, and now it appears that our mental health has also been affected. Dr. Martin Seligman[1] suggests that our new Western lifestyle is resulting in alarmingly higher rates of depression and that depression is striking us at much earlier ages. He cites two studies which show 10- to 20-fold increases in depression in America during this century. One investigation revealed that people born after 1945 are 10 times more likely to suffer depression than those born 50 years earlier.

Incidence of major depressive disorders has shown a steady gradual increase over the course of this century. People born around the time of World War I (who have had a great deal of time to get depressed) show rates of only about 1 percent. Those of us born around 1925 show rates of 4 percent, those born around 1960 have rates of 6 percent, and those born more recently have major depression rates of 8 to 9 percent. A second epidemiological study discussed by Seligman revealed depression rates which were 20 times higher in people born after 1950 than in those born prior to 1910. Seligman believes that modernization of cultures results in greater passivity and feelings of helplessness, hopelessness, despair, and low self-esteem. Other, less westernized cultures show no such consistent trends, and suicide and depression are completely unknown in some primitive cultures.

An interesting finding has emerged from a recent study of the Amish people in Pennsylvania. This group of farmers manages to cling to a mid-19th-century way of life in which electricity, automobiles, and other labor-saving devices have no place. Rates of bipolar depression, which are largely the result of inherited genetic defects, are the same among the Amish as in other areas of America. But Amish rates of other depressions, which are more sensitive to social forces, are only one-fifth to one-tenth the rates seen in other areas of this country where we have become more modernized.[2,9,10]

While the Amish have totally maintained a mid-19th century lifestyle, some rural areas of America have resisted rapid urbanization more than others. One such area is Stirling County (a pseudonym) in Canada. This county was quite rural at mid-century and has moved rather slowly toward small-scale urbanization in the ensuing twenty years. It was the site of large-scale mental health surveys in 1952, and again in 1970. Rates of depression and anxiety disorders showed no change between 1952 and 1970 in a large representative sample of more than 2000 men and women in that area.[8] We shall see in a later chapter that mental disorders are related to urbanization.[9,10]

Depression appears to be associated with both where and how we live. A recent occupational stress survey[11] of a large group of American men and women has revealed that depression was positively related to increased recreational drug use and to increased time spent in front of the television set. On the other hand, depression was negatively correlated with sport participation. People who engaged in physical play tended to be less depressed than those who sat in front of TVs or smoked dope. While these findings don't imply cause and effect, depression does appear to be associated with sedentarianism and the television habit.

Certainly the low rates of depression among the Amish reflect a very large number of cultural influences, but two things which the Amish culture most definitely does not include are TV sets and labor-saving devices.

The Good Life has come to be an unnaturally sedentary one, and now we see a flood of scientific data pouring in from many diverse disciplines, data which underline the centrality of physical activity for human well-being. These data suggest that regular exercise is required to fulfill our genetic design specifications for normal, trouble-free functioning.

While many aspects of the Good Life can impact both physical and mental health, this book focuses largely on the psychological consequences of an unnatural sedentary lifestyle. Even at this early juncture in scientific research, there is enough consistency in the findings of experiments which explore the relationships between exercise and mental health to warrant our attention.

Before examining these research findings, let's take a look at some Americans who do exercise regularly and see what they have to say about why they began and why they persist. Just exactly who are they, and why have they turned their backs on a way of life where even walking is largely unnecessary?

Chapter 2

The Pathfinders

Paul Spangler packed his sweats and went to Israel in the spring of 1987. There he would represent the USA in the International Masters Track and Field Games. *Masters* translates into everyone 40 and over. In Israel, Paul competed in the 3000 meters on a Friday. He raced in the 5000 on Saturday. On Sunday he ran the 10,000. He won three age-group gold medals. During the final ceremonies, 600 athletes from around the world stood and sang Happy Birthday to Paul. On that day he had turned 88.

A week later Paul stood and talked with me after a race on the Stanford University campus. Paul's time that day was well off his effort in the previous year's race. He conceded that he hadn't fully recovered from his Israel effort. He was also thinking that he would have to lay off racing for a couple of months and do some alternative training in order to allow a persistent hamstring problem time to clear up. He wanted to be in first-rate shape for next summer's world games in Australia. He was after another marathon record.

Paul was lean and lucid. So were the other men and women who raced that morning in California's brilliant sunshine. It was the annual run of the Fifty-Plus Runners' Association, a group of about 1500 men and women who are committed distance runners over the age of 50. The organization's basic purpose is research, and members serve as subjects in a wide variety of studies on the physiological and psychological effects of regular distance running on older men and women. They, quite incidentally, also serve as an alternative lifestyle model in an aging culture.

Once a year the members get together for a seminar, an annual meeting, and a race. The race is an unusual one by most standards since the age-group categories begin at 50 and continue at five-year intervals up to 100. Race times that day ranged from 30 minutes to about an hour for the hot, five-mile course. Not bad. Some raced fiercely that morning, inviting the sort of sustained pain which competitors of all ages endure when running just below the red line. Others ran easily, simply celebrating health, life, and fellowship. Everyone was in good shape. You could tell, because they were all breathing quite normally just moments after crossing the finish line. Vital and good-humored, they looked 10 to 20 years younger than their actual ages. Spectators who wandered by and chatted with course workers were amazed to discover that these men and women were all over the age of 50.

What unnerved the spectators about these chronologically "older" men and women was that their behavior seemed so very appropriate and natural. They were, in fact, "acting their ages," for all of them possessed relatively youthful cardiorespiratory, skeletal, and muscle systems—not to mention attitudes strikingly different from the sort you see in retirement communities. For example, let me share a communication from one of the members. She is a 60-year-old Californian who has run more than 40,000 miles since she began at age 40. I had asked her to summarize her reasons for running on a postcard. She wrote,

> I can't remember why I began, maybe to curb a tendency to overeat, that plus the determination to live to be 140 and buy it on downhill skis. I continue for all of the obvious health benefits—to be able to have my cake and shed it too. In spite of some really bad things which have happened to me in the past few years, I remain relatively sane. My sanity may not be attributable to running, but I am unwilling to test that possibility. The same thing is true for arthritis. I am convinced that running keeps it in check. I remain flexible and pain-free. Finally running enhances my view of myself. I value myself more thinking of myself as an athlete. I am a runner.

I am certainly not suggesting that everyone should model themselves after this extraordinary, vital woman. What she significantly offers us is an alternative way of living which she has found has many benefits. More importantly, she exuberantly flings open two doors which have been closed for far too long. She lets us know that it is all right for women and older persons to exercise and think of themselves as athletes.

When compared to other older men and women, the people who raced that day were certainly unusual. But it is important to know that before they began to exercise regularly, they weren't particularly special people—just your ordinary generic *Homo sapiens sapiens*. Many, like Paul, didn't buy their first pair of running shoes until they were in their 60s. Some began long before.

Even when the seductive sun of the Good Life had reached its zenith during the warm and lazy days of the 1950s and 1960s there were those who had turned away. They were the scattered and isolated pathfinders of what would become a new tribe, nonconforming men and women who independently turned their backs on the toxic elements of the Good Life to explore a faded trail which their bodies confirmed was right. While epidemiologists were busy clarifying the relationships between how we lived and why we died, these early pathfinders had already assumed primary responsibility for their own physical and mental health.

Often we were in bed when they were about, but on occasion we caught glimpses of them. The ghostlike silhouette of a single scull silently carving the early mist and gray water of the Charles River. The distant, distorted figure of a hunched-down cyclist slowly taking shape through the heat waves shimmering over a two-lane Kansas blacktop. The reed-thin, wavering shadow of a distance runner flowing with the spreading sunlight through the rolling vineyards of the Napa Valley.

Back in those days we tolerated them, but not always with good grace. They were difficult to understand. Perhaps they sensed that it was hopeless to expect sedentary people to understand, since they seemed to have little interest in explaining themselves. They simply went on doing their particular thing.

Sedentary psychiatrists and psychologists wisely explained that these daily rain-or-shine physical rites were compulsive and masochistic, the manifestations of paranoid tendencies, perhaps male anorexia, or veneers which thinly concealed deep depression. While sitting at lunch troweling mayonnaise on their arterial walls, social scientists speculated that these strange and solitary exercise-eccentrics were acting out midlife crises, denying their mortality, and clearly not acting their ages. Observing their long odysseys, we perceived them as lonely rather as simply engaging in a solitary activity. We thought them social misfits who were running away from the problems of real life—problems which we more stalwartly stood and faced. It was difficult for us to see their daily rituals as a responsible way of dealing with life.

Being a pathfinder was tough. However, we can forgive ourselves for reacting to them as we did. We don't like to be reminded of our mortality, and these people held a mirror before us which made us uneasy. Whether it is love or hate at first sight, we always react with our strongest emotions to those people whose behavior mirrors things about ourselves which we prefer not to admit. It is always tough to get around to admitting that we would be better off if we were somewhat more like the people who upset us the most. In the eyes of these early pathfinders we saw reflections of our soft flabby bodies and the potentially lethal consequences of our self-indulgent and indolent ways.

While the pathfinders weren't keen on being seen as pathological sneaker freaks, they were not the sort whose behavior was much predicated on social approval. They persisted, and as time went by more and more people turned their backs on the Good Life and joined their ranks. Exercise is now respectable. Sweat has become fashionable. Even those of us who are largely sedentary wear costumes which suggest that we are on the way to or just returning from a bout of exercise. We go shopping about town in our high-tech sneakers, leg warmers, head bands, and designer sweats—the sort of stuff most regular exercisers wouldn't be caught dead in. For them training has always been a very private affair.

The Primitive Contemporaries

Epidemiologists sometimes classify this emerging tribe of primitive contemporaries as the LANS, the Lean, Active Non-smokers. Barring an accident, or the bad luck of having been dealt a poor genetic hand, LANS people not only will outlive most of us, but will remain unusually healthy, active, and fit during their entire lives. They will visit doctors less often than most of us and will be relatively immune from the chronic diseases which make so many of us infirm and dependent in our autumn years. They will redefine what it means to act our age. While we are struggling with chronic lower back pain, emphysema, osteoporosis, cancer, or the consequences of a first heart attack, LANS people old enough to be our parents will be running marathons. Little wonder that they make us uneasy.

The Fitness Boom

Just who exactly are these LANS people? Why are they so persistent, and why did they start doing the things they do? For starters, estimates of their numbers have been exaggerated. The great fitness boom is more like a modest bang. Only 15 to 20 percent of Americans exercise enough to maintain even minimal cardiorespiratory fitness. ·A recent 21-state survey by the Centers for Disease Control indicates that more than half of us don't exercise enough for even minimum health benefits. The most bleak figures come from the southeastern states, where around 70 percent of us are sedentary. In 1984, when about 40 million of us solemnly swore to George Gallup, Jr., that we were running every day or nearly every day, a careful in-depth survey suggested otherwise. American Sports Data found that only about 12 million of us ran regularly at about that time, and of that group slightly more than a million ran more than 40 miles each week.

Those Who Were Left Behind

The fitness boom hype perpetuated by magazines created to cash in on the swelling tide of athleticism suggested that the nation was flooded with newborn athletes, and that people of all ages and from every walk of life were riding the wave. Not true.

Runners may not represent a cross section of sport participants in America, but I am going to talk about runners here because of the wealth of information available concerning them. American runners are almost exclusively white, and mostly male. While athleticism has become acceptable and even desirable for women of late, their numbers have leveled off and account for only about 20 percent of runners. The old and the young are also minorities. Few are younger than 20 or older than 60. Most are between 30 and 50 years of age.

Blue and White Collars

Runners are mostly well-educated, reasonably affluent, white-collar professionals. One survey tells us that the highest percentage are educators (more than 1 in 10), followed by doctors and dentists, engineers, and accountants. Within business and industry, those who hold management positions are more likely to exercise. Blue-collar membership has risen slowly over recent years but seems to be holding at about 15 percent. Big business would like it otherwise. Painfully aware of the swelling corporate costs incurred by the consequences of sedentary lifestyles, many have built on-site fitness centers and provide a variety of health-promoting programs for employees. But even where participation is encouraged, it is the Yuppies who predominate. The reasons are several.

Some of it has to do with scheduling. Men and women who hold management positions, as well as various other professionals, purchased their scheduling freedom by spending long expensive years at colleges and universities. Now finished with their training, they have considerable flexibility in setting up schedules which will accommodate blocks of time for exercise, cooling down, and showering during workdays—certainly more flexibility than the men and women on the production line. Professionals and management people can frequently shift schedules when changing daylight hours and seasons dictate. Educators at all levels typically have summers off, and self-employed professionals have infinite flexibility. So while the corporate fitness centers might invite everyone to dance, the blue-collar worker can't always fit it into his or her program. The blues have rigid schedules and must periodically switch shifts, a process which insults circadian rhythms and generally makes life more difficult.

Education

The management people and professionals who are more likely to exercise regularly are also better educated than blue-collar workers. Perhaps this translates into keeping better informed and taking greater personal responsibility for well-being. For example, since the 1964 Surgeon General's Report on Smoking, there has been a high correlation between education and quitting. Today 20 percent of college graduates, 30 percent of high school graduates, and 37 percent of high school dropouts smoke. But correlations do not imply cause and effect. Some other factor or factors could be responsible for certain of us both pushing on through school *and* not smoking.

Personality

Personality is certainly a significant factor which might have a great deal to do with predicting whether or not we are likely to make regular exercise a part of our lifestyle. It also has a role in predicting what sorts of exercise we might prefer.

Some of us who have incorporated regular exercise into our lives have chosen physical activities which, to the outsider, appear to be repetitious, boring, and lonely. Day after day, and month after month, certain of us swim lap after boring lap or run mile after solitary mile. Some of us not only do boring repetitious things, but we train on days when we don't feel like it, when the exercise doesn't feel good, when we are mildly ill or injured, and on days when adverse weather keeps most others inside.

Others of us chose social games which involve varying degrees of competition. We like to be around people and have fun while we work out. These sorts of stop-and-go sports such as basketball or tennis are exciting and can distract us from our daily worries. They also often include important team bonding and support.

Solitary *aerobic* endurance activities such as swimming and running attract different kinds of people and offer different sorts of rewards and benefits from stop-and-go social games such as volleyball or racquetball.

Let's take just a moment before going on to clarify what is meant by "aerobic" exercise. *Aerobic* literally translates to "with air," so aerobic exercise involves an intensity sufficiently moderate to allow us to replenish our oxygen as we continue to work out.

Sprinting, on the other hand, is anaerobic (without air). We use more oxygen than we can take in during such periods of intense effort and incur "oxygen debt." We have all had the experience of being "out of breath" and had to slow down or stop. Discontinuous activities such as tennis and basketball, which are characterized by brief, intense bursts of action, are generally considered to be anaerobic and less effective in building cardiorespiratory fitness. *Aerobic exercise requires a significantly increased amount of oxygen over a sustained period of time, not so much as to incur oxygen debt, but enough to result in increasing our cardiorespiratory fitness.* Aerobic exercise has a cardiorespiratory "training effect." The standard measure of cardiorespiratory fitness is $Vo_{2_{MAX}}$ (*maximum oxygen uptake, the maximum volume of oxygen we can breathe in and deliver to our working muscles in a given time period*).

While regular aerobic exercise can increase our $Vo_{2_{MAX}}$, other forms of vigorous exercise, such as weight lifting, may result in muscle development with no significant increase in our cardiorespiratory fitness. Cardiorespiratory fitness is most often increased with "endurance training" or "aerobic" activities such as sustained swimming, running, bicycling, very brisk walking, and aerobic dance. I will talk more about these concepts later on, but let's get back to a discussion of what sorts of people are more likely to choose these aerobic forms of exercise which have such important physiological benefits.

Personality and Delay of Gratification

As children, what we experience within our families can shape our personalities in very significant ways. For example, some of us had parents who provided consistent consequences for our positive and negative behaviors, and who allowed us to experience healthy frustration. They didn't allow us to manipulate them and they didn't solve our problems for us. Consequently, we learned early that there were significant personal rewards if we could tolerate frustration, figure things out for ourselves, and delay our gratification. Add to that learning to take responsibility for our behavior, and we were well on the way toward self-sufficient, independent adulthood. Parenting of this sort might predispose us to being able to incorporate healthy aerobic exercise into our lives.

While many of us have histories of doing without and waiting, not all of us actively chose to invite or prolong these agonies. Future professionals do. Some put off marriage, children, financial security, and all sorts of spiffy material things for 10 or more years of college and internships. Once done, they have a great deal of independence and flexibility in their lives. The final awarding of a university diploma testifies to things learned, but it also certifies that the recipient is an independent, responsible, and persistent sort—the sort who can tolerate frustration and delayed rewards. Graduate school is a little like training for and successfully completing a marathon or swimming the English Channel.

While our experiences can substantially shape our personalities, we each arrive in life as the product of a unique genetic package which predisposes us to behave in particular ways no matter how much our parents and society might wish to otherwise shape us. Any parent who has had more than one child will swear that each was different from the others from Day 1.

Boredom Suseceptibility and Need for Change

Some of us, for example, are risk-taking, uninhibited, and adventuresome seekers of new experiences, people with little capacity to tolerate boredom. We may have sisters or brothers who are quite the opposite. Marvin Zuckerman[7] has devoted his life to the study of "sensation seeking" and is convinced that it is an adaptive universal human trait. He also argues that there is some reason to believe that it may, in part, be biochemically and genetically determined.[8] Not all of us have an average or optimal need for change, but such a need has obvious adaptive and survival value. Some of us have far too much or unusually little need for change, and that can create problems. Those of us with an unusually high need for change may take too many risks and suffer injury or even death. On the other hand, those of us with a subnormal need for change might get left behind, facing whatever consequences that may bring. We are not all created equal with regard to sensation-seeking needs. Let me give you a couple of examples.

A few years ago a parachuting friend of mine was given the task of coaching the Norwegian National Alpine Ski Team. *Alpine* translates into breathtaking and dangerous high-speed slalom and downhill racing at speeds up to nearly 100 miles an hour. Like other high-risk sports, alpine skiing attracts a certain breed, a breed very different from those who are drawn to cross-country ski racing. My friend, thinking that these downhill racers should increase their endurance (cardiorespiratory fitness), prescribed mandatory daily jogging. The whole team quit. They preferred to ski for fun and not to go to the Olympics rather than have to suffer the boredom of jogging. As time went on my friend realized that they were dead serious and had to give up on the jogging.

But even sensation seekers have many dimensions. For example, the average total score on Marvin Zuckerman's Sensation Seeking Scale V is about 22 for young men aged 16 to 20, and scores gradually decrease with age, down to about 13 for men my age. I score at 28. I mention these numbers for two reasons. One is to suggest that no matter what our need for change and sensation seeking, for most of us it diminishes with age. This could mean that some of us who cannot tolerate the boredom of aerobic exercise in youth might find it to be quite acceptable when we have grown older. The reason I include my rather aberrant score is to underline the fact that not all of us are average or normal, and that our personalities are very complex. Even a personality factor such as sensation seeking has many dimensions. For example, I score high on subscales which measure thrill, adventure, and experience seeking, but very low on a subscale which assesses boredom susceptibility. Thus, I was twice blessed. While answering an inner summons to pursue a life filled with sensation and experience seeking, change, and adventure, my capacity to tolerate boredom allowed me to spend nine years working my way to an advanced degree, and further blessed me with being able to run every day.

Now that we know that there are different forms of exercise with different payoffs, and that they might attract different sorts of individuals, let's talk some more about who exercises and who does not.

Those Who Drop Out

Historically, those of us who would benefit the most from regular exercise either don't begin or, if we do, quickly drop out.

The most predictable dropouts from fitness programs are those of us who smoke, those who are overweight, and, interestingly enough, those of us who are poor credit risks. While wearing out credit cards, smoking, and overeating may seem like diverse behaviors, they have at least one important thing in common. The thread of immediate gratification weaves its way through them all. Blue-collar workers who shun company fitness facilities and programs are also conspicuously absent from company programs aimed at weight reduction and smoking cessation. While the Yuppies work out at lunchtime, others are more likely to be found in the cafeteria—sitting, eating, smoking, and talking about installment purchases.

The Motivation of Distance Runners

LANS people come in all sizes and shapes, and they engage in all sorts of activities. But the differences between them are quite superficial. Regardless of silhouette, they tend to be lean. Lean does not refer to our shape, it refers to the percentage of our weight that is lean body mass rather than fat. Another thing which they share is that when they are asked about why they exercise with such persistent regularity, the predictable reply is simply, "It makes me feel good." For the uninitiated, this unrehearsed and spontaneous answer makes sense if the response comes from a tennis player or even a bicyclist. But to hear it from those who engage in solitary and seemingly dull endurance activities such as lap swimming or distance running seems to raise more questions than it answers.

A Pilot Study

It was nearly a decade ago that a number of scientists from Stanford and San Jose State Universities helped organize the Fifty-Plus Runners' Association, and when we put together our first newsletter I invited our 400 fledgling members to take part in a pilot study which inquired about their reasons for running.[3] There were all sorts of expert opinions around at the time, but precious few data on what motivated men and women to exercise regularly for years on end. The newsletter included a long checklist concerning commonly stated reasons for beginning to run, a small group of current motives to be ranked, and a checklist which concerned what people thought about when they ran.

Our average female member at that early juncture was 55 years old and had been running about 24 miles a week for four years. The average male was 57 and had been running about 35 miles a week for eight years. These people took their exercise seriously, and I figured that what they had to say had to count for something.

I discovered that most of these men and women had begun to run because of a concern about cardiovascular and general physical fitness. Having lived more than a half century, most were well aware of their mortality. They had taken over primary responsibility for their physical and mental health, choosing to enhance both the quality and the quantity of their remaining years.

Many had begun to exercise with regularity after losing a father, husband, or brother to a heart attack or stroke. Losing a close friend or family member to a heart attack when he is relatively young can be sobering indeed. More than 1 in 10 of the men began to exercise on a doctor's orders to control high blood pressure. Being directly told that unless we lower our blood pressure we could suffer sudden death as a result of a cardiac event causes us to take pause and consider how we are living.

Part of the fitness concern was focused on weight control. One-third of the men and one-half of the women checked this as a significant factor in motivating them to begin regular exercise. Comments from both men and women made it clear that the weight concerns reflected motives associated with physical health, attractiveness, and self-esteem.

Of significance was the finding that a fourth of the women and a fifth of the men had begun to run to find relief from depression and anxiety. Many were depressed as the result of loss. Death, divorce, and separation were frequently mentioned. A substantial number of the women had begun to run as a reaction to the depression and identity crisis precipitated when left with an empty nest. Suddenly all of the children were gone and life had lost some of its meaning. The longtime meaningful role of mother was no longer needed. Running had helped these women through a rough period until new roles and meaning were established. It had similarly helped many men get through the difficulties associated with retirement or job loss.

Just as many of these men and women had begun to exercise to cope with depression, an equal number had begun running to control tension and anxiety which were generated on the job or were the result of domestic problems. Some exercised in the morning to immunize themselves from the tension they knew they would encounter at work. Others relieved the day's accumulated tensions by running after work. A 59-year-old man wrote me that he had begun to run in order to find out "what it was all about" but quickly adopted daily running because it helped him get rid of what he called the "AWFs," which turned out to be his anxieties, worries, and frustrations. He related that some mornings he woke up feeling simply "AWF-full."

Another important psychological factor concerned personal identity or self-concept. Four questionnaire statements which were commonly checked were "I needed space, privacy, and time to be alone," "I was tired of fulfilling everyone else's needs," "I was tired of being defined by others and fitting into the mold," and "There was no longer anything in my life that belonged only to me."

When it came to ranking the current motives which importantly sustained regular running, the number-one-ranked item for both men and women was "Maintaining a strong, trim, healthy body." Two important psychological payoffs were tied for the second ranking. They were "The psychophysiological release and energization *following* each run" and "My new independent identity as a runner." The word *following* is emphasized here because one of the significant discoveries in this pilot study was that these men and women seemed to exercise more for its *effects* than for the rewards they experienced while actually running. Thus the fact that the joggers we see alongside the road often look miserable may be quite irrelevant to the scheme of things. A statement concerning the psychophysiological release experienced while running and another concerning competition got the lowest rankings.

My conclusion was that the motives of these runners focused on three central, but not completely independent, motives. First and foremost were concerns about physical fitness, weight control, and longevity. The other two central motives were psychological: the first concerned exercising to regulate moods and anxiety, and the second had to do with enhancing identity or self-concept. A fourth, less significant, motive concerned running to regulate social distance—to satisfy needs for privacy or social contact.

I used this pilot work to develop the Runner Motivation Test. It was later revised for use with men and women who engaged in a wider variety of aerobic activities and was renamed the Test of Endurance Athletes' Motives (TEAM). The two tests were nearly identical, and a copy of TEAM is included in the appendix. Definitions of the motives have been slightly modified (the words *regular exercise* have been substituted for *endurance training*) so that if you exercise in any manner at all, even simply walking regularly, you might want to turn to the appendix and take the test yourself. Then you can read on and see how your scores compare with those of other men and women I have tested.

The motives used in the studies we will be talking about are listed below. *Fame and Fortune* was used on the original Runner Motivation Test, since that test would be administered to some world-class professional runners. It was replaced by *Addictions* in the TEAM test which was used with an older group of athletes.

Addictions: To stop or control antilife habits such as smoking, drinking, or drug use through regular exercise.

Afterglow: The elevated mood and reduced tension which *follow* regular exercise.

Centering: Space to be alone, to clear my head, and to simply experience myself and the world around me. The *psychological experience while exercising.*

Challenge: To challenge or gradually improve myself through participation. To gradually perform better than I did in the past.

Compete: To challenge others and to define myself in relation to other competitors.

Fame and Fortune: To make money and/or a name for myself as an athlete.

Feels Good: The various *rewarding physical experiences while exercising.* The exercise itself feels good to me.

Fitness: The cardiovascular and general physical fitness which *follows* regular exercise.

Identity: The independent definition of or statement about myself: I
  exercise. I am an athlete. It is my lifestyle.
Slim: To control weight and appetite through regular exercise.
Social: To meet new friends or to be with old ones through exercise,
  competition, or club activities.

The *Running Times* Study

I struck a deal with the editors of *Running Times* magazine and
was able to get more than 700 of their readers to take the original
Runner Motivation Test.[4,6] The men and women ranged from early
teenagers to senior citizens, but nearly 70 percent of the men fell
within 10 years (above and below) of the average age of 38, and a
similar percentage of the women fell within 8 years of the average
age of 35. The men had been running an average of about 40 miles
a week for about 6 years, and the women had averaged about 34
miles a week for about 4 years. Serious runners.

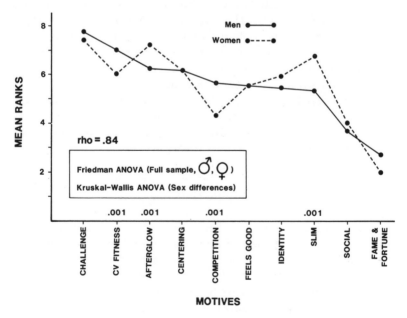

Current running motives for 700 experienced male and female distance runners.

The first thing that impresses me about the results of the testing is that the relative strengths of the various motives were very similar for both men and women. The positive correlation of .84 is very high indeed, but there were some differences. The small numbers at the bottom of the figure represent statistical confidence levels, the odds that the differences we see on the preceding page are attributable to chance. The .001 below competition, for example, tells us that the odds are only 1 in 1000 that the difference between men and women was due to chance. We can be quite sure that the men were more competitively motivated than the women. Where there are no small numbers below a given motive we can assume that whatever sex differences we may see are chance differences.

The men in this group were more concerned with physical fitness, were more motivated to compete, and were more concerned with making a name for themselves through running ("Fame and Fortune") than were the women. The women, on the other hand, were more motivated than the men to run for the emotional state which followed running ("Afterglow") and for weight control ("Slim"). The overriding conclusion, however, is how very similar the motive strengths were for the two sexes. Fitness, for example, was a stronger motive for men than for women, but it was also a very important motive for women. The same is true with regard to "Afterglow" for the men.

There were a few other things about the motives of this group of runners that were noteworthy. Challenge to self was a very strong motive for both sexes, but the motives concerned with social needs and fame and fortune were very weak.

Aerobic Dancers

Barbara Edmiston, one of my undergraduate students at the university, was interested in how the motives of the female runners might compare to those of women who did another form of aerobic exercise. She found 100 regular aerobic dancers, women who had worked out at least three times a week for a year, and gave them a slightly modified version of the Runner Motivation Test.[2]

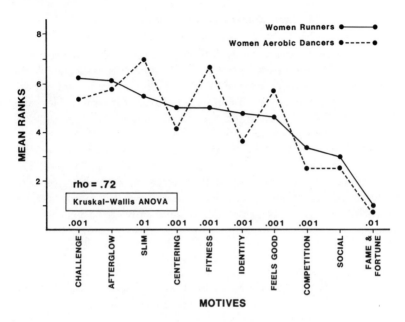

Motives of 150 experienced women distance runners and 100 regular women aerobic dancers.

While there is an impressive positive correlation between the motives of the women who ran and those who danced regularly, there are significant differences in motive strengths on 8 of the 10 motives. The aerobic dancers had stronger motives with regard to fitness and weight control, and it appears that aerobic dancing must also feel better than distance running. No surprise there.

The women runners were more motivated to challenge themselves and to psychologically center themselves while exercising. They were also more competitive, more concerned about identity, and more strongly motivated to make a name for themselves. They appeared to be a different breed of cat, maybe a little tougher and more competitive. But when compared to world-class professional women marathoners, these women runners were pussycats. The pros were tigers.

Elite Woman Marathoners

I was able to test a group of the best women distance runners in the world some years ago during the Avon International Women's Marathon series. Some of these women had competed in past Olympics and others would compete in future Olympics. Here we see the motives of these highly select women along with those of our other very serious women runners.

The primary motives of this group of elite runners were all centered on winning. Their strongest motivation was to challenge themselves, and in this regard they were no different from the nonprofessional women runners. But beyond this single shared powerful motive, they appeared to have only three very strong motives: competition, identity, and fame and fortune.

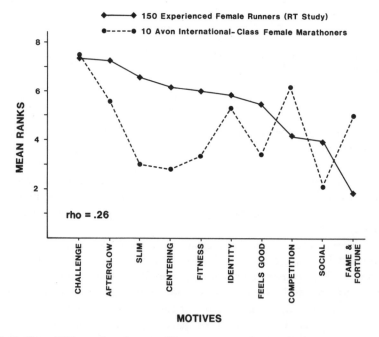

The motives of 150 experienced women distance runners and 10 world-class women marathoners.

The other motives which count importantly for less talented runners were very likely taken for granted by these world-class runners. These women had only around 10 to 15 percent body fat and were obviously not concerned with staying slim. To put that into perspective, the other highly fit female runners would have had body fat percentages mainly in the very low 20s, and similar women who were normally inactive would have had percentages in the low 30s (about 17 percent body fat is considered ideal for men, while percentages in the low 20s are considered ideal for women).

The world-class women marathoners were also unconcerned with fitness. They were already off the top of the charts on all such dimensions.

Finally, it looks as though running didn't feel all that good to the professionals. Not hard to understand if you think about having to run 65 to a 100 or more quality miles week in and week out for years on end. Competition can take the fun out of things for many of us.

It also looks as if the motives of these elite runners were not social ones: they didn't run to be with other people. They got together with their competitors on occasion to try beat them. The rest of the time they trained.

Age, Experience, and Changing Motives

I found myself wondering whether the motives which started people running were the same ones which kept them running year after year. Could the strength of these various motives change with experience? Might we begin to exercise for one or two compelling reasons and then discover other significant reasons after we had exercised regularly for months or years? Having a rich data source in the Fifty-Plus group, I decided to do a retrospective (looking-back) study. I gave some of our members the TEAM test with directions to take it once within the framework of why they now ran, and once again with regard to why they began.[5]

Nearly 200 men and women took part, with the men outnumbering the women five to one. The men averaged about 56 years of age and had been running about 10 years. The average woman was

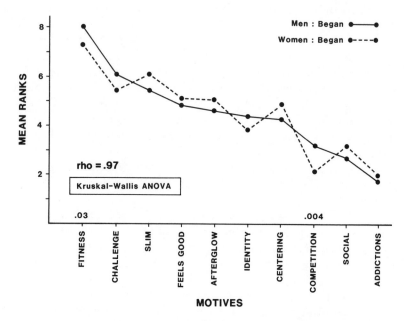

Initial running motives for 200 experienced older distance runners.

about 53 years old and had been running about 6 years. Both men and women were currently running about 25 miles a week. Women who have run 7000 miles and men who have run 14,000 should have something of value to say about motivation.

The results reveal that these men and women, who mainly had begun to run when middle-aged, had remarkably similar motive profiles. The correlation is very high indeed, suggesting that the relative strengths of the motives which got these men and women started running were very similar.

As in the case of the *Running Times* study, which involved men and women who had lower average ages, the men had significantly higher motives than women with regard to both physical fitness and competition. However, these older male and female runners ranked fitness (rather than personal challenge) as the strongest motive for beginning to run. This group also ranked weight control as a more important motive (the women ranked it as

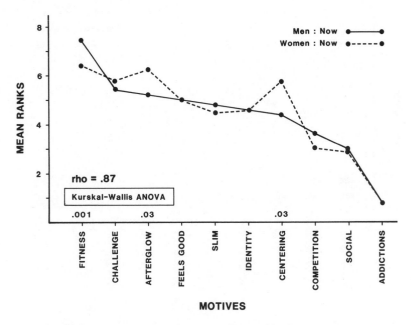

Current running motives for 200 experienced older distance runners.

second strongest), and they also relegated competition to a lower position. Addictions' very low ranking reflects the fact that it was an initial motive of concern to only a small percentage of the group.

When we look at the current reasons for running, the most obvious feature once again is that the motive strengths for men and women were parallel. The similarity is very striking. The men remained more concerned with fitness than the women, but the early difference between the two sexes with regard to competition had disappeared. What is of special interest is that two psychological motives now differentiated the two sexes. It appears that the psychological centering experience while running and the postrun mood elevation and tranquilizing effect of exercise had become significantly more important for the women as running experience continued. Let's have a look at the specific motivational changes that occurred for men and women as running became incorporated into their lifestyles.

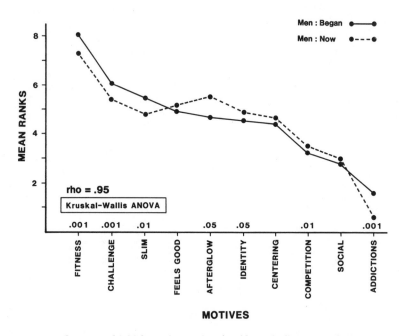

Current and initial running motives for older male distance runners.

Men's motives for beginning to run and their motives for continuing to run showed similar relative strengths. Nonetheless, there
were significant shifts in the strengths of 7 of the 10 motives. While
fitness, challenge, and weight control remained very strong motivating factors, they all significantly decreased in strength. This shift
might reflect that these initial goals had been achieved and the gains
were more taken for granted. It is of significance that psychological
motives became stronger with experience. The mood-elevating and
tranquilizing postrun payoffs from running become more important
for men with running experience, and the increased strength of
identity may reflect a change in self-esteem which had resulted from
having achieved a major change in health and lifestyle.

The significant drop in addictions suggests that those men
who began to run in order to give up or control tobacco and alcohol
dependencies were no longer concerned about them. I received
autobiographical statements from all of the men and women in this
group, and it appears that of the entire group, only a single woman

had failed to give up the addiction (to tobacco) which had motivated her to take up running. Her story was a strange one. She began to run when in her late 50s, and discovered that she had harbored a great athletic potential. Before long she became an ultramarathoner, regularly competing in races longer than the standard 26.2 mile marathon. But she complained that instead of losing her cigarette addiction, she now had two addictions. She related that she carried cigarettes in a fannypack during 50-mile mountain races, and that when she stopped for a break she would light two cigarettes at once in order to save time when inhaling an energizing hit. I sometimes wonder if she is still alive, what with subjecting her heart to such peril. At any rate, she was an anomaly. The rest of the men and women who had begun to run in order to kick alcohol or nicotine dependency made it. This is also seen in the changes in the women's motives.

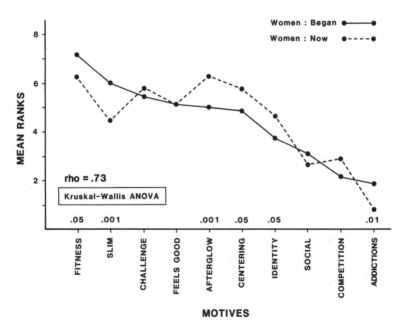

Current and initial running motives for older female distance runners.

The shifts in motive strengths that were revealed by the men were dramatized by the women. The women told us that the early concerns about fitness and weight control which had got them started running had decreased in importance, and that the psychological rewards had significantly grown in importance with running experience.

While both the men and the women increasingly ran for psychological benefits as their experience built, these motives appeared to be somewhat more important for women. My pilot study on a larger sample of older runners suggested that a substantial number of women began to run to ease depression and anxiety, and the results of this later work underline how much more compelling psychological motives become when women discover how effectively running can impact their moods.

Pulling the Studies Together

Taken together these studies suggest that the compelling motives for regular distance-running fall into three categories. We run

1. For cardiovascular and general fitness
2. To feel good (mood and anxiety control)
3. To feel good about ourselves (self-esteem)
4. Another very central motive, weight control, is involved in all three of the other categories.

These findings are very similar to those of two other investigators who administered questionnaires to 315 men and women a few years earlier. Carmack and Martens[1] reported that the runner's perceived outcomes of running were:

1. Physical health (cardiovascular conditioning and weight control)
2. Psychological uplift (decreased anxiety and improved mood)
3. Self-image (self-respect, sense of identity)
4. Affiliation (fellowship with other runners)
5. Achievement (success in competition)

Carmack and Martens also found that psychological uplift, or running to feel better, became more important with running experience.

Most of us begin to run to get in shape. Men and women alike are looking for cardiovascular fitness, firm muscles, strong bones, and lean bodies. More men than women become heart attack statistics quite early in life, and that might account for fitness being a slightly stronger motive for them. However, it was also the Number 1 motive for beginning to run for the older women I studied. Two other powerful reasons for beginning to run, to challenge self and to control weight, are equally strong for both sexes.

The business of losing and controlling weight being of equal importance to men and women is not surprising in an America where percentage of body fat can sometimes play a complex social or even political role. Both men and women associate being thin with being attractive to acquaintances, friends, sexual partners, and even employers. But apart from these psychological factors, there is a much more significant reason for such concern. America is a dangerously overweight country, and as we put on increasing weight we put ourselves at greater risk for a host of life-threatening conditions. Preoccupation with thinness does have pathological dimensions in a very small percentage of our population (less than 1 percent), but male and female distance runners are not a pathological group, and they tell us that they want to lose weight for health, to feel better about themselves, and to look both sexy and attractive. Other things being equal, the closer we can approach our ideal lean body weight, the healthier and longer-lived we shall be.

The Shift toward Psychological Rewards

As men and women settle into regular running, the relative strengths of their important motives begin to change. Fitness remains the Number 1 motive for both men and women, but along with weight control, it becomes less important. Being lean and fit become taken for granted—accomplishments which will persist as a part of a new lifestyle.

As miles begin to add up and weeks roll by, psychological benefits are realized and become central motives. These increasingly strong motives have to do with how we feel about ourselves and with how we feel, our emotional moods. They become basic in sustaining regular training for both sexes.

Longtime runners concur that building well-conditioned, lean bodies is usually accompanied by increased self-esteem. It is of significance that the means to the end may be as important as the end itself. While a lean and fit body is a satisfying end product from a long exercise program, the independent engineering process itself provides a sense of internal control that can create a sense of self-sufficiency which is almost priceless: "No doctors. No pills. I did it. I know how. I could do it again."

Regular endurance training can also provide a source of identity, the knowledge that in addition to whatever else we may be, we are athletes. This private knowledge is a little like wearing a Superman or Wonderwoman shirt under our regular duds. Ask the other people on your block if they can run 10 miles, and they will likely ask if you're insane. Ask LANS, and the answer will be, "How fast?"

As we get hooked on regular exercise, it becomes more important. The *it* in that sentence is an important one. The late Dr. Fritz Perls, who founded Gestalt psychotherapy, always insisted that we not objectify ourselves in his presence—that we always say *I* in place of *it*. Think about it. "It doesn't matter" can translate into "I don't matter." At any rate, when "it" (regular exercise) becomes more important, the "it" is actually ourselves. We begin to matter more. When we begin to exercise every day, insist that an hour of each day belongs to ourselves exclusively, and tell others that they will have to somehow adjust their needs and expectations to allow us our exercise period, we're making a strong statement about ourselves: "My running is important. My time is important. My needs are important. I am important."

Our self-esteem and identity are also tied into the personal challenge which physical endurance activities offer. People who never dreamed they could ever run an single mile might one day hike the entire length of a mountain range, run a marathon, or bicycle from coast to coast. Realizing an athletic potential which has been dormant all of our lives can serve as a powerful metaphor and springboard for other things in life. We may find the courage to set vocational or educational goals which in the past might have seemed impossible. We each dwell within our own personal arenas, and the challenges to take risks and to attempt the intimidating or impossible are always there waiting for us.

Personal challenge is a primary motive for people who exercise regularly, be they beginners or elite Olympic stars. What's more, challenging ourselves is remarkably different from competition as most of us have experienced it. This difference is very apparent in foot racing. On any given weekend, one finds such races scheduled across the country. They can be "fun runs," timed races, or a combination of the two. The distances are typically 5, 8, or 10 kilometers (about 3, 5, and 6 miles). There may be anywhere from a few hundred participants on up to more than the 100,000 that run San Francisco's famous 7.4-mile "Bay to Breakers." It is not difficult to figure out that most entrants in such races are not elite runners. These races are for everyone.

In a typical weekend race, those runners who are pushing hard against their limits are almost always challenging themselves rather than attempting to defeat other people. They use other runners and the emotion-generating power of the race to pull themselves along toward a personal best, a personal record which they could almost never achieve on a solitary run. Runners typically view other runners, not as people to be defeated, but as comrades who help one another be more courageous than they could possibly be by themselves. A footrace mostly involves running with other runners rather than against them.

While there are few trophies in a distance race, there are many winners. Any person of any age who can simply finish such a race at any speed is a winner. During a given race many people will pin a number on their shirt front for the very first time and will worry about being the last to cross the finish line. Some will run a race distance farther than they have ever attempted before. Some will put forth supreme effort to run the distance faster than they have ever done before, and others, whose times are well off their personal best, know that in spite of great adversity, their efforts were heroic.

For me, simply finishing a marathon is a heroic act, what with having a distribution of fast- and slow-twitch leg-muscle fibers which suggest that my ideal racing distance is a single mile. But of the many marathons I have run, the three heroic efforts, the ones which can bring back tears and powerful images, were all more than a full hour slower than my fastest. One was run on an unforgiving, cloudless, blistering, and humid day, when in spite of drinking as often as I could, I lost nearly 15 pounds. During another, I dealt with enormous broken blisters and bleeding feet the last 10 miles. The most memorable was a race where I suffered intestinal cramps and diarrhea the last 20 miles. If you have never willingly subjected yourself to such adversity, it is very easy to dismiss such behavior as being stupid or pathological. Perhaps so. But this rather bland and civilized world rarely offers us these affirming personal tests of character. I seem to periodically need to do something heroic, and to be reminded that I possess courage and inner resources far deeper than are ever demanded or experienced in everyday life.

But most races are not marathons, and most efforts are not heroic. People go to such races to enjoy themselves. My very first race taught me some important things. First of all, I didn't have to worry anymore about coming in last. It probably would never happen, and if it did, people would very likely applaud me for simply finishing. I also found the other participants to be exceptionally friendly and supportive, rather than competitive. Most importantly, I learned that there were people of all ages, sizes, and descriptions who could beat me. I remember an incident about a mile from the finish during my first race. I had found some hidden resources and had picked up my pace, passing people rather steadily. I was giving it my best effort when this young girl in a wheelchair pulled slowly up on my right. I stayed with her for a couple of blocks, then shook my head, smiled at her, and waved her on. These footraces are celebrations of fellowship, vigorous health, and life.

There are, of course, some runners for whom competition is important. They are few, mostly male and mostly young. However, the vast majority of distance runners are after other things. Challenging ourselves is a whole different ball game from attempting to beat everyone else. It offers good stuff for everyone, rather than empty trophy cups for the few. Giving it your best is not the same as being best. Personal best is not best.

Exercise and Mood Control

A couple of years ago I spent a cold spring May Day Eve in Kringsjå, a university student community on the outskirts of Oslo.

I was drinking beer and talking about life with a student. He and I had met quite accidently but had become instant friends, only discovering later that we had both stood on the same mountain peak in Asia, and that we had both spent some time in free-fall. He was an expert parachutist. I had just commented that I always felt that I had returned to my home planet each time I visited the Norge Idrettshøgskole (the Norwegian National Sports College), where faculty and students of all ages routinely exercised every day. Trond looked out into the black foggy night and, without forethought, quite seriously replied, "Yes, if we could not exercise each day, we would all be mad."

Athletes routinely and offhandedly make reference to this relationship between sanity and endurance training. For example, when world-class endurance swimmer Julie Ridge was asked by *Sports Illustrated* why, as a freshman at Boston University, she had begun to swim a mile of laps each day in the tiny university pool, she replied, "It was a sanity thing."

Besides making us feel better about ourselves, regular exercise makes us feel better. It does this in two important ways. One has to do with the centering experience which occurs while actually training. The other has to do with the emotional afterglow—the post-workout tranquilizing and mood-elevating effects. Let's start with centering.

Existential Drift

Many of us prefer to exercise by ourselves, not because we find it difficult to relate socially to others, but instead, because we need relief from it. Social interaction of all kinds is stressful. For example, simply saying "good morning" to a close friend results in an increase in blood pressure in both people.

Solitary walks, runs, and swims allow us to get centered, to clear our heads, and to simply experience ourselves and the world around us at a very elemental level. When we are infants, our thought processes are "primary" images and associations based on contiguity and common elements, rather than the more logical, causal, rational sorts of "secondary" processes which come with the development of language. As adults we engage in both sorts of thought processes. For those of us whose lives are ruled by "secondary" processes, exercise offers a situation to leave such sometimes headache-provoking processes behind.

Aerobic exercise always involves rhythmic, repetitious, almost hypnotic movement resulting in a significant increase in our body core temperature, much like that produced in a sauna or hot tub. The almost magical interplay between energization and relaxation produces a sort of primitive meditative state where our awareness is frequently focused almost exclusively on our body and our immediate physical environment.

Without the protective shell which a building or automobile provides, walkers, runners, and bicyclists can feel the weight of the humidity, the steepness of the mountain, the rush of the wind, the drifting odors, and the sting of the raindrops. This sort of precious existential drift, this immediate and elemental here-now awareness, provides relief from the stresses of the social world. It is the most common mental state which distance runners report and seek, and it probably accounts for the fact that we see so very many of them on solitary journeys, and why we often see them outside on stormy days. This sort of existential drift has a way of putting things into perspective—of reminding us of just what matters and what does not. Being in touch with our bodies and the world around us, robust good health, feeling good, and the magnificence of simply being alive are things which matter. Against this backdrop, the crisis at the office and the new dent in the Mercedes fender have little meaning.

Unfocused existential drift was the most common kind of mental activity which men and women in my pilot study reported experiencing when they ran. The second most common activity was a focus on breathing or running technique, an almost meditative state. From this rather primary and elemental state came the spontaneous upwelling of creative thoughts, the third most commonly reported mental activity. Solutions to what seemed like unsolvable problems, or the dramatic organization of material which seemed previously chaotic, often burst into consciousness when we are fully concentrated on nothing more than making it up to the top of the ridge.

A California composer, 65-year-old William Kraft, reports that when he runs into a compositional impasse he puts on his running shoes and heads out on a 45-minute run up into the Angeles National Forest. The problems seem to work themselves out on the trail.

I prefer to start my days with a morning run, but when I am at work full time on a writing project, like Kraft, I do my best composing in the morning. By early afternoon persistent mental fog predictably moves in and begins to cloud my thinking. Then, like Kraft, I, too, go for about a 45-minute run. It is then that I do my best work. I run in an attempt to clear my head and find relief from my work, but throughout the run my mind will unpredictably drop in and out of my writing for short moments. What is so interesting about this is that the creative process which is involved will very often focus on sections of the manuscript which I worked on days or weeks before. The first thing I do after a postrun stretch is pick up a pencil and jot down the ideas which came while running.

I know a large number of Silicon Valley engineers and others who work in research and design in computer-related facilities, men and women who also run each day. So very many of them, like Kraft and me, have independently discovered that the best of all times to run is during their noon lunch breaks, after a sometimes frustrating morning of work. All sorts of solutions to work problems seem to come forth spontaneously when these men and women are doing nothing more than trying to forget them.

As in the case of so many other important things which we seek, giving up trying is often the solution. Constantly seeking the approval of others, putting all of our efforts into finding Mr. or Ms. Right, or obsessing about a difficult work problem, all these things can get in the way of finding what we seek.

Besides the centering experience and creative wellspring which exercise provides while we are actually working out, it also seems to importantly affect how we feel afterward, elevating our moods and reducing our anxiety between bouts of exercise.

Depression and Anxiety

There are times when unrelenting depression will not yield to medication, psychotherapy, the support of good friends, or prayer. At these times some of us, as a last resort, turn to sneakers.

It is our hope that the pain which hard physical training inflicts on our out-of-shape bodies will distract us from our obsessive ruminations, ease our anxiety, bring relief from black depression, and grant us sleep. The testimony of thousands of runners says that these hopes can be realized.

The pain of such last-resort running can temporarily take our minds off our problems. Even the pain of sore muscles can lend a hand over the next 24 hours. The run can also give us relief from our anxiety and help us find sleep. Once realized, postrun mood elevation becomes a central motive. There is a saying among runners, a kind of fundamental truth which all old runners take for granted: "No depression can stand up to a 10-mile run."

Little wonder that we see sneaker freaks running along the roadsides in blistering heat, torrential downpours, darkness, and bitter cold. Little wonder that they go through withdrawal and become impossible to live with if illness or injury interferes with their daily medication.

Some of us exercise in the morning to immunize ourselves from the day's inevitable stresses. It's hard to get upset about things when our muscles feel as if we just stepped out of a sauna and our heart is kicking over 20 beats a minute below normal. Some of us exercise in the evening as a form of therapy, to clear the day's tensions, elevate their moods, and relax for a good night's sleep. During tough times, some do both.

Sudden changes in exercise behavior sometimes signal personal crises or periods of stress. When someone begins to focus more on training schedules, distance, speed work, racing, and the like, friends suspect that there may be trouble in paradise. Thus, from a mental health standpoint, we might view exercise in terms of routine preventive dosages which help us tolerate routine stress and ward off depression, and periodic heavy dosages to enable us to weather the really tough periods.

We can all become obsessive when things begin to fall apart for us, concentrating our obsessions on one aspect of our lives to avoid having to deal with what is really the matter. For example, some of us become workaholics, alcoholics, or concerned parents and focus on those issues to avoid worrying about more significant problems such as a marriage which is dying. A sudden increase in exercise frequency or intensity might help us to cope with stress in a healthy way. It could also serve as a maladaptive distraction from having to confront urgent and important issues.

Controlling Addictions

A large number of the men and women I studied had begun to run regularly in order to control weight. A smaller number had begun to run with the hope that it might impact their addiction to cigarettes or alcohol. While many reported that running helped them to kick one or another addiction, there is no real, hard, documented evidence on this. At least two large surveys on runners show that about 50 percent previously smoked and that about 3 percent of the women and 1 percent of the men continued to smoke after beginning to exercise with regularity. However, the cause-effect relationship is blurred. It is common for ex-smokers to say that as they increased the number of miles they ran each week, they reached a point where they had to give up either running or cigarettes. Other runners report, "I stopped smoking and started running," suggesting that some other strong motives set up a readiness to do both. While it has yet to be demonstrated that fitness programs can effectively impact smoking, it has been demonstrated that smokers are very likely to drop out of fitness programs.

Social Motivation

While social motivation may sustain participation in some sports, it does not appear to be an important motive for the runners I studied. Even the small percentage of runners who belong to organized running clubs run alone most of the time. Some important benefits can only be realized alone.

It seems hard to believe that the raucous, high-energy, rock-and-roll atmosphere of an aerobic dance class isn't a highly social experience, but the social motivation of these women appears to be no stronger than that of female distance runners. Aerobic dance might offer some social support. A commitment to meet a friend and drive to workouts two or three times a week, or experiencing the support of other people working out with them, might have something to do with getting the women to keep coming to sessions. But the activity itself is something else. Once the music starts and the familiar routines begin, the dancers appear to go on automatic pilot and get into their own private, centered state.

But dancer or runner, the core motives remain the same. Those of us who engage in aerobic endurance exercise regularly seek physical fitness and weight control; we want to feel good; and we want to feel good about ourselves.

Testimonials about the many benefits realized by mature men and women who have logged tens of thousands of miles simply cannot be ignored. The big question now is whether or not there is any scientific support for their claims. Does research confirm that endurance training increases longevity, provides immunity from heart attacks, builds strong bones, and helps control weight? And how about mental health claims? Does exercise really tranquilize anxiety, reduce depression, and enhance self-esteem?

Our major concern here is with mental health. So let's begin with a look at those psychological disorders that most commonly trouble us, and let's consider what causes them. Then we will check out the effectiveness of the current chemical and psychological treatments of choice (preferred or most effective) for these disorders. Then we will see how exercise stacks up when faced off against these more conventional treatments.

Chapter 3
American Angst

Americans are a troubled people. At this moment, one out of every five adults, about 29 million, suffers from some form of mental disorder. In the course of our lifetimes one in three of us will so suffer.

Men and women who suffer from schizophrenia roam through the canyons of our inner cities. They live beneath our bridges and in our doorways. Now that we have closed down so many of our mental health facilities, they frequently inhabit our jails. But high-exposure and sometimes dramatic disorders such as schizophrenia, and eating disorders such as anorexia, are relatively rare in contrast to those which trouble most of us.

A recent landmark National Institute of Mental Health (NIMH) epidemiological study of mental disorders in America has in many ways eclipsed all earlier attempts to survey mental illness in this country.[21,25,26] More than 17,000 people in five communities were individually interviewed in this $15-million investigation, and the findings paint the most accurate picture of the incidence of mental disorders in America that has ever been available.

The NIMH interviewers used the American Psychiatric Association's definitive *Diagnostic and Statistical Manual of Mental Disorders (DSM-III)*[8] as its source of diagnostic categories, and as a result, some old assumptions have been laid to rest. Previous surveys had, for example, consistently found women to be more psychiatrically disabled than men. But earlier investigators had never inquired about alcohol and drug problems, or about antisocial personality problems. The NIMH people finally did, and they concluded that men and women have similar lifetime mental-disorder rates. The "Good Ol' Boy disorders" just didn't used to count.

One of the other interesting new findings was the surprising prevalence of anxiety disorders. This category includes disorders such as phobias, panic attacks, and obsessive-compulsive disorders. Depressive disorders were thought to be the most common mental problems in this country, but the NIMH survey discovered that about 8 percent of us suffer from anxiety disorders, and that they constitute the most common group of psychological problems which trouble Americans.

The NIMH team found that the next most common group of disorders was substance abuse and dependency. Between 6 and 7 percent of us are afflicted. Alcohol dependency accounts for about four out of every five cases. The best figures predict that during our lifetimes between one in six and one in nine of us will abuse or become dependent on alcohol. These are astounding numbers. The obvious drunks on skid row constitute a tiny minority, only about 5 percent of alcoholics. Most of us with alcohol problems flow in the mainstream of society. We raise families, work, and drive on the freeways, where we are responsible for more than half the deaths and injuries.

Americans also become addicted to certain activities, such as gambling and persistent overeating, and these addictive behaviors mimic the substance dependencies. Their etiologies and behavior patterns are very similar to those of substance dependency, and they share a resistance to treatment. While thought of as personality disorders (rather than substance abuse disorders), they are serious and widespread.[33]

Depressions are also common. Quite apart from the uncomplicated normal depressions which all of us suffer from time to time, about 1 in 20 of us will have to contend with a severe major depression during our lifetimes. Depressions constitute the third most common group of disorders in America. They afflict about 6 percent of us.

The NIMH researchers, who prided themselves on including the Good Ol' Boy disorders in their recent survey, did not bother to mention America's most prevalent mental disorder. It's included in the DSM-III chapter on substance abuse. Tobacco dependence is hands down the most widespread and the second most lethal of our mental disorders. Alcoholism afflicts 10 to 15 million adult Americans, and alcohol ranks (after coronary heart disease and cancer) as the third most common cause of death in this country. Tobacco dependence still afflicts more than one in four of us and accounts for an astounding one in every six deaths in this country.

The millions of us who still smoke are obviously neither insane or suicidal, but with the grave diggers quoting such lethal odds, those words do have a certain ring to them. Those of us who smoke die sooner from just about every fatal disease. Racing motorcycles, skydiving, and mountain climbing, are remarkably safe and sensible activities when compared to voluntarily smoking cigarettes.

Gender and Mental Disorders

It should be no surprise to learn that the NIMH people discovered that men and women deal with stress in different ways. Science frequently simply adds credence to what we already knew to be true. When women are overstressed they are more likely to develop different kinds of disorders from men. They are also more likely to seek help.

The NIMH researchers found that 57 percent of the men and 75 percent of the women who had suffered from recent DSM-III disorders had visited a mental health provider.[28] A recent NIMH survey of patients who visited psychiatrists and psychologists in private practice revealed that 40 percent of patients were men and 60 percent were women.[35]

We will see that a wide variety of biochemical, psychosocial, and sociocultural factors predispose men and women to various sorts of mental disorders. Men in our culture, for example, walk in the collective long shadows of John Wayne and Rambo. Men also model themselves after those bumbling but lovable ex-jocks who make the TV commercials about the Big Beer Brotherhood of Men, commercials which drum out the message that sports and athleticism somehow go hand in hand with drinking. When tough guys get depressed or anxious, they are more likely to medicate themselves with alcohol. Tough guys don't need help.

Alcohol has, for centuries, been the male nonprescription treatment of choice for tension and the blues. Alcoholism was a problem during the Golden Age of Greece, and both wine and beer made the Dark Ages a little less dark. Then about 800 A.D., when the Norse were building exotic rowboats, generally running amok, and definitely making England much less jolly, an Arab alchemist discovered the process of distillation. Alcohol has historically provided chemical courage to soldiers facing death, and a drink or two has always served to loosen the rest of us up in tension-producing, but less potentially lethal, social situations. As Ogden Nash commented, "Candy is dandy, but liquor is quicker." Whether mixing in cocktail parties or bedrooms, liquor has a way of making things easier. A couple of beers with a buddy after work have always quieted the dragons generated by bosses and wives who don't understand.

While alcoholism has long been considered a male disorder, alcohol abuse appears to be growing among women, and the commonly quoted estimate of one female to every five male alcoholics is considered conservative.

It has been recently discovered that alcohol impacts a particular neural system (the GABA-benzodiazepine receptor complex) with the identical marvelous tranquilizing effect of a prescription benzodiazepine such as Valium.[34] Little wonder that heavy doses of Valium are widely used in detox units to ease the pain of alcohol withdrawal. And if alcohol is a kind of cheap, over-the-counter Valium, little wonder that alcohol can frequently emerge as the identified problem for many of us, masking whatever it was that precipitated our drinking in the first place.

Men have significantly higher rates of alcohol abuse and dependency than do women, and it's highly likely that they also have higher rates of drug abuse and dependency. Men also get rowdy and write their own rules more often—their rates of antisocial personality disorders are far higher than those of women. When men go for treatment, it is most likely to be within a substance abuse program.

Women, on the other hand, have higher rates of depression and various sorts of anxiety disorders. They have clearly higher rates of major depressions and both agoraphobia and simple phobias. It is very probable that women also have higher rates of minor depression, panic attacks, obsessive-compulsive disorders, and schizophrenia. They are also more likely to convert their anxiety into recurrent and multiple bodily complaints—complaints for which there is no real physical disorder. I will be describing what sorts of symptoms characterize these various disorders shortly, but let's first finish looking at the picture of mental disorders in this country.

Other Demographics

Essentially the same overall lifetime mental-disorder rates hold not only for men and women, but also for blacks and whites, and for people in various sections of the country. Everyone, however, is not at equal risk.

Those of us between 25 and 44 years of age suffer the highest overall mental-disorder rates. Perhaps these are the most stressful years for most of us. College graduates have significantly lower overall mental-disorder rates, and perhaps because they are more likely to continue to actively use their heads, they have lower rates of cognitive impairment when they grow older. Drug problems afflict mainly the young, those in the 18 to 24 age group.

Overall rates of mental disorders increase with urbanization. Rural areas have lower overall rates of mental disorders than urban areas and specifically have lower rates of drug, alcohol, and antisocial personality disorders than urban inner cities.[26]

If we set aside the lifetime picture and take a look at what troubled Americans during a typical six-month period during the present decade, the most common disorders for men were alcohol abuse and dependency, and the most common disorders for women were phobias and depression. Here again, disorder rates drop sharply after the age of 45. The most recent analysis of the data which came from this landmark study reveals that 15 percent of us suffer from substance abuse or other mental disorders each month.

The stability of disorder rates may vary as a result of several factors. For example, bipolar depressions which have clear genetic bases might occur with considerable consistency over time and across cultural subgroups, while other depressions which have more clearly psychogenic bases and are more responsive to stress might be more variable. Chapter 1 suggests that depression has dramatically increased during the course of this century.[6]

We are going to focus largely on the depressions and the anxiety disorders in this book. One reason is that they are so common here in America. The other reason is that the vast majority of research on exercise therapy has dealt with the treatment of anxiety and the mood disorders. This is precisely because exercise appears to be most effective in the treatment of these two classes of mental disorders.

The Anxiety Disorders

The anxiety-based disorders are the most common disorders which afflict us, and they include what used to be called the neuroses. Freud considered the neuroses unconsciously learned maladaptive behavior patterns, efforts to cope with excessive anxiety which was generated by unacceptable impulses which created conflict within us. This diagnostic group includes somatoform disorders such as hypochondriasis and conversion disorders. The term *somatoform* refers to a category of mental disorders where physical symptoms suggest physical disorders, but the disorders actually have no real organic basis. They are psychologically based. Hypochondriasis involves preoccupation with fears or beliefs of having a serious disease, and a conversion disorder involves a loss or alteration of physical function such as blindness or paralysis which is rooted in psychological conflict rather than organic pathology. Anxiety-based disorders also include the more rare dissociative disorders, such as amnesia and multiple personality where individuals deny responsibility for their behavior and avoid stress by escaping from their core personality.

While many disorders have anxiety components or bases, one group is officially classified as anxiety disorders. We are going to concentrate on this group. These disorders, which are characterized by irrational and unrealistic fears of an intensity sufficient to sometimes disable us or make us nonfunctional, are the most common mental disorders in America. Women suffer higher rates of panic disorders and the various phobias, but obsessive-compulsive disorders afflict both sexes with similar frequency.

Panic disorder is characterized by recurring unpredictable anxiety attacks. While these attacks normally last only a few minutes, they are terrifying. The physical symptoms are the same as we all feel when we are frightened, but they are so intense and bewildering that we may fear dying, going crazy, or completely losing control. Anticipatory fear of helplessness and loss of control can increasingly restrict us to the safe haven of our home. When we begin to avoid public places for this reason, we suffer from agoraphobia with panic attacks.

The essential feature of *agoraphobia* is irrational fear of being alone, or being alone in public places where escape might be difficult or help might not be readily available in case of an emergency. The situations most commonly avoided are crowds, busy streets, elevators, crowded stores, tunnels, and public transportation. Those of us who suffer from agoraphobia frequently won't leave home without a family member or friend.

Simple phobias involve a fear of particular situations or objects such as enclosed places, heights, or animals. Once again, they are more prevalent among women. Phobias which begin in childhood often disappear without treatment, but those which persist into adulthood normally require treatment.

Less common are *social phobias*, where the essential persistent and irrational fear is of situations where we may be exposed to scrutiny by others. Speaking or performing in public causes most of us anxiety, but phobic individuals are more incapacitated and are likely to avoid such circumstances. Even simple acts such as eating or writing in public can be traumatic for the individual with irrational fears about being exposed to scrutiny.

Obsessive-compulsive disorders are quite widespread in America, affecting 2 to 3 percent of us.[24] These disorders involve uncontrollable involuntary thoughts (obsessions) or behaviors (compulsions) which we are unable to control. Obsessive thoughts, images, or impulses seem to penetrate or intrude into our consciousness despite all of our efforts to ignore or suppress them. We think of them not as being products of our consciousness, but rather as foreign invaders.

Examples of compulsive behaviors include such things as hand washing or rigid routines (which are repetitively carried out according to certain rules) which are experienced as involuntary.

We cannot resist giving into them, and they seem not so much to have a realistic and sensible end as to affect some future event or situation. It is as if the happening or nonhappening of some future event hinges on our carrying out these rather senseless routines. Certainly our anxiety hinges on doing so, because when we act out the behavior, we experience a release of tension. But once acted out, the tension begins to build again, eventually pushing us to repeat the behavior. Obsessive-compulsive disorders can seriously interfere with how we function both socially and on the job.

Those of us who suffer from obsessive-compulsive disorders are commonly depressed. The two disorders appear to be related biologically and both respond to similar medications. At this point researchers don't know whether obsessive-compulsive disorders are a form of depressive disorder, cause a secondary depression, or are the result of a primary depression. Whatever the case, they overlap.

Finally, some of us suffer from what is called a *generalized anxiety disorder*. If you can remember how you felt when you experienced stage fright, you have an idea of the sort of persistent symptoms involved in this disorder. In addition to periodic sweaty palms, racing heart, dry mouth, shaky knees, dizziness, and trembling hands, individuals with such a disorder experiences worry, rumination, apprehension, difficulty in concentration, sleep difficulties, fatigue, jitteriness, and irritability. Not a pleasant package to have to predictably deal with.

The Mood Disorders

Normal Depression

We all have our ups and downs. We all go through periods of feeling discouraged and sad, sometimes feeling helpless and hopeless about the future and despairing that we may never feel better. At such times we often feel unusually dependent, self-critical, and ineffective. But most of our depressions seem to be self-limiting and come to an end almost irrespective of what we do. We frequently feel stronger and better off for having coped with and survived a depression which at times seemed as if it would never end. Depressions often serve a useful purpose, forcing us to face and work through problems we might otherwise avoid. We are sometimes surprised at the ease with which we can let go of a depression, when it has seemed as if it would last forever.

Normal depression is predictably tied to some sort of identifiable environmental stressor. Grief or loss is perhaps the most common cause. The loss can be job-related (we lose a job, are transferred to another city, fail to get promoted, or retire), can involve separation (leaving home, moving away from a best friend, a failed romance, or a divorce), or can involve the death of a pet or someone you love. The grieving process has been well documented and normally takes about a year to work through.

We also commonly experience depression when we finish something very important. Reaching a significant goal sometimes feels anticlimactic. The outcome doesn't quite match up with the investment, effort, and anticipation. Perhaps this is yet another form of grieving. Examples include the letdown which about half of women experience after childbirth or the depression that comes when we are awarded our diploma after years of college or postgraduate work.

Periods of depression are quite normal. It is when our depressive reactions go beyond the normal boundaries of frequency, duration, and intensity that we suffer from a mood disorder.

The Less Severe Mood Disorders

Some of us suffer from mood swings, periodic excesses of elation (hypomania) and depression. When down, we may be unable to sleep or cannot stop sleeping excessively. We have no energy, lose interest in pleasurable activities such as sex, and often withdraw into a tearful, brooding, and pessimistic state. The hypomanic (moderately manic) periods are characterized by behaviors which are opposite those of the depressed phase. These consist of rather frantic optimistic times when nothing can bring us down and we don't even seem to need sleep. It is the unpredictability of these periodic mood swings, which interrupt otherwise rather normal functioning, that identifies us as suffering from *cyclothymia*.

Our mood can swiftly change for no apparent reason. Cyclothymia may well be a mild form of the much more serious bipolar disorder which we will discuss shortly.

If we suffer from long periods of depression with symptoms like those of the down period of cyclothymia, but without ever going through hypomanic phases, we suffer from *dysthymia*. This is a kind of chronic moderate depression which lasts for years, punctuated occasionally by brief periods of normal functioning which may last only for days or weeks, seldom for months.

In addition to cyclothmia and dysthymia, the DSM-III includes another form of moderate depression under the category of adjustment disorders. *Adjustment disorder with depressed mood* differs from dysthymia in that it has a clear cause which has stressed the individual and in that it doesn't last as long (no more than six months). The depression differs from normal depression in that the individual has overreacted to the precipitating cause, and in that the depression interferes with his or her social and vocational functioning. This depression, as you might suspect, is a tough one to call. Just where normal begins and ends gets hazy when it comes to evaluating just exactly what is an appropriate reaction to circumstances and events which stress us.

The Severe Depressions

Cyclothymic and dysthymic disorders have more severe counterparts which are called *bipolar disorder* (at one time referred to as manic-depressive disorder) and *major depression* (unipolar disorder). These disabling disorders appear to involve biological defects which predispose us to periods of profound mood disturbance which do not require an environmental trigger. Their symptoms differ from those.of cyclothmia and dysthymia largely in terms of duration and severity.

If we have suffered even a single manic episode, we are diagnosed as bipolar, although there is evidence that a few of us might suffer periodic manic episodes without depressive periods. When in a manic period we become extremely active, talkative, restless, irritable, and distractible. We may have racing thoughts, flights of ideas, and inflated self-esteem and sometimes do foolish, impulsive things. Some of us, during manic periods, become psychotic, hallucinating and having delusions which frequently have themes of inflated worth and power. We usually have our first episode in our late 20s, and about 60 percent of us who suffer such an episode will have recurrent episodes throughout our lifetime.

The symptoms of major depression are largely exaggerations of those which characterize dysthymia. However, they can assume very serious proportions. We can become preoccupied with thoughts of death and suicide, lose interest in eating, and begin to lose weight. Sometimes we suffer from hallucinations and delusions which have very depressive themes, or we fall into a depressive stupor where we become so unresponsive that, if left alone, we fail to eat and perish. These sorts of deep depressions more commonly recur, and while figures vary considerably, it appears that more than 60 percent of us who suffer from major depressions will have recurrent episodes (with an average length of about four months) throughout our lives. Between depressive episodes our lives are understandably compromised.

The Search for Causes

Our Stone Age ancestors were no doubt troubled by mental disorders. Psychotic behavior has very likely been around for as long as we have. During prehistoric times, shamans (primitive medicine men) searched for the causes and cures for bizarre behaviors. They settled on evil-spirit possession as the cause, and on trephins (circular holes in the skull: evil-spirit escape hatches) as the cure. I expect the shamans both prevented and cured a certain number of mental disorders. Even the prospect of having a hole cut in one's skull with a sharp rock could have powerful effects.

With the advent of Christianity, evil spirits came to be seen as demons or agents of the Devil, and getting rid of them became the responsibility of the clergy. During the Middle Ages, religious exorcism of demons was the primary treatment for the mentally ill. However, during the 16th and 17th centuries, diagnostic and treatment techniques became excessive. Torture was the diagnostic device, and the cutting out of tongues, beheading, and burning at the stake became the solution for tens of thousands of diagnosed heretics and witches. Mental illness was perceived as God's punishment for sin, or as the result of deliberate association with the Devil. These notions concerning the causes of mental illness dominated thought until well into the last century. From our distant beginnings up until very recently, the consequences of madness were grim. But now, after 30,000 years of evil spirits and exorcism, humanism has prevailed and the search of the causes and cures of mental disorders has fallen into the hands of scientists.

By early this century scientists offered both physiological and psychological explanations for disordered behavior. Physicians demonstrated that brain pathology, such as that caused by syphilis, resulted in dementia, and early social scientists, such as the psychiatrist Sigmund Freud in Austria and the psychologist J. B. Watson in America, demonstrated that behavior disorders could also be the result of experience and psychological conflict.

Genetic Factors

Twin studies and studies of adopted children have long suggested a genetic basis for both bipolar and unipolar (major depression) disorders, and the bipolar disorders appear to have an even stronger genetic component than do the major depressions. The bipolar concordance rate for fraternal twins (percentage of the cases where both twins have the disorder) is 14 percent, and for identical (monozygotic) twins the rate is 72 percent. The respective concordance rates for unipolar major depression are 11 and 40 percent.[1] Very recently, after years of having to infer genetic involvement from such studies, a genetic marker has been discovered.

Dr. Janice Egeland and her research team have studied the small, contained Amish community in Pennsylvania, where they were able to document cases of bipolar disorder going back for several generations within particular families. These researchers identified a genetic marker for bipolar disorder on the short arm of the 11th chromosome. Sixty-three percent of the Amish people carrying this genetic defect showed bipolar symptoms.[9]

The fact that women suffer more frequently from major depressions as well as agoraphobia and panic disorders, and that all of these disorders have been impacted with antidepressant medication, has caused some researchers to speculate that there might be an X chromosome genetic factor involved. Two studies on mother-daughter and father-son concordance rates suggest that this hypothesis might be a tenable one, but a final answer awaits future research.[23,38]

In 1988 two investigations were reported which shed light on the biogenic factors involved in schizophrenia. One research group that studied five large Icelandic and two large English families found a genetic marker, or susceptibility locus, on chromosome 5 of the 39 schizophrenic individuals in those families.[29] A second group, who studied northern Swedish families, found no such marker on chromosome 5 of those schizophrenic individuals, suggesting that different genes may be responsible for schizophrenic susceptibility in different families.[15] Dr. Eric Lander, who reviewed these two studies, suggests that a gene on chromosome 5 may represent only a minor cause of schizophrenia and points out that schizophrenia is not entirely genetically determined since the concordance rates of the disorder are only 50 percent among identical twins.[16] But he sees the research as significant in that it reveals that at least some cases of schizophrenia are monogenic, predisposed by a single gene.

The discoveries that schizophrenia and bipolar disorders have genetic and biological bases should help to reduce the social stigma associated with individuals who suffer from these disorders.

Neurochemical Factors

Up until very recently the relationship between our behavior and the neurochemical events within our brains has been largely a mystery—our brain an inaccessible black box. But space-age technologies, which were undreamed of only a few decades ago, have opened previously locked doors and have allowed neurochemists to begin to explore the biological aspects of mental disorders.

Scientists have discovered that *particular areas of the brain and particular neural pathways form systems which are associated with various mental processes such as pleasure, pain, depression, anxiety, and organized thought. Each of these systems utilizes particular neurotransmitters, chemical messengers which relay signals across gaps (synapses) between neurons within the system.*

It is important to take a moment and describe what happens at synapses, and how messages travel along neural systems. The electrical energy which terminates at the end of a presynaptic neuron releases neurotransmitters which travel across the synaptic gap and briefly bind onto specific receptor sites on the postsynaptic neuron. These receptor sites will accept only that particular kind of neurotransmitter. Thus the neurotransmitters are like keys which will fit specific locks. If enough neurotransmitters bind onto receptor sites, the presynaptic message will be transmitted to the postsynaptic neuron and continue to travel along the neural pathway. It's an all-or-none process. A postsynaptic neuron either fires or it does not fire depending on the presence of a sufficient number of neurotransmitters. We shall see that the number of these neurotransmitters available at synapses along certain neural pathways are related to our moods and can be affected by things such as drugs and exercise.

These chemical messengers actually do more than simply transfer messages. They can also influence the activity of other neurotransmitters. When they perform that function, they are referred to as *neuromodulators*. The same chemical regulators may operate as hormones (*neurohormones*) and travel in the bloodstream to influence systems distant from their point of origin. Our interest will be in their role as neurotransmitters, and the neural systems which utilize the neurotransmitters dopamine, norepinephrine, serotonin, and beta endorphin are of special interest to us. These systems constitute only a small fraction of the total number of neurons in our brains, but they are important because of their central role in emotions, thought processes, and behavior disorders, and because their activity is also influenced by exercise. Let's begin with a consideration of some of the many ways in which these four neurotransmitters may influence our behavior.

Dopamine

Excessive dopamine synaptic activity, an excess of dopamine receptors, and supersensitized dopamine receptors have all been hypothesized as biological factors involved in schizophrenia. The "dopamine hypothesis" rests on the results of postmortem examinations which reveal excessive dopamine receptors in areas of the brain which mediate emotion and thought processes,[17] on the fact that a paranoid schizophrenic state can be produced quickly in any of us by an injection of amphetamine (which floods our brains with dopamine),[30] and on the fact that antipsychotic medications which dramatically reduce schizophrenic symptoms do so by blocking dopamine receptor sites.[7]

One problem with the dopamine hypothesis is that the effectiveness of the antipsychotic medications is not limited to schizophrenia (they also effectively treat psychotic symptoms in some manias, in organic mental disorders, and in toxic disorders resulting from drugs such as LSD). Another problem is that these remarkably effective drugs block receptor sites within hours, but symptom relief may require days or weeks. More recently it has been suggested that low levels of two particular hormones, one of which is associated with an enzyme which breaks down dopamine, may play a role.[37] Whatever the solution to the questions concerning the biochemical causes of schizophrenia, an overactive dopamine system plays an important role.

Dopamine insufficiency, on the other hand, is associated with Parkinson's disease. Antipsychotic medications which reduce schizophrenic symptoms by blocking dopamine activity will induce Parkinsonian symptoms, which, in turn, must be medicated. On the other hand, medication which increases dopamine activity in Parkinsonian patients can produce schizophrenic symptoms in some of them. One expert suggests that all of us are walking a dopamine tightrope, with too little leading to Parkinson's disease and too much leading to schizophrenia, and that in some of us the safe range is a very narrow one.[4] This makes it very difficult to medicate those Parkinsonian patients who are predisposed to schizophrenia.

Dopamine also appears to have a role in depression. In the next chapter I will discuss how both antidepressant drugs and the bipolar medication lithium appear to affect dopamine receptors in our brains. Dopamine plays a critical role in the pleasure centers of the brain, and dopamine system adaptation is very likely central in individuals who abuse amphetamine (speed) and cocaine. Finally, above-average levels of dopamine have been related to extraversion.

Serotonin (5-Hydroxytryptamine)

A large research effort is now focused on the neurotransmitter serotonin. It appears that serotonergic systems are involved in a broad spectrum of behaviors. A glass of milk and a cookie before bed, for example, work as a sedative for many of us. Both the milk and the cookie can influence serotonin levels in our brains, and serotonin plays a central role in wakefulness and sleep. A lower midbrain structure called the *raphe nuclei* is rich with neurons which utilize serotonin. Mild electrical stimulation of this area produces sleep, and destruction of these neurons results in insomnia.

Dairy products, such as milk and cheese contain considerable L-tryptophan, a large amino acid which is a chemical precursor (used in the synthesis or manufacture) of serotonin. When levels of L-tryptophan are raised in our blood, the chances of more of it passing through the blood-brain barrier (a biochemical filter which regulates what substances pass between our blood and brain neurons) to be converted to serotonin are enhanced. Health food stores do a big business in L-tryptophan because it is such a fine sedative. It's very effective but does not have the addictive, potentially lethal, or extended aftereffect qualities of prescription drugs. When taken at night, prescription drugs are still in our systems and active the next day, leaving us groggy and impairing our performances. Even state-of-the-art benzodiazepines such as Xanax are only half out of our systems by morning, a problem for layover airline pilots who sometimes use benzodiazepines to get sleep in a new time zone.

The serotonergic system is also sensitive to diet in a more general and ancient way. Drs. Judith and Richard Wurtman of the Massachusetts Institute of Technology have carried out research which suggests that serotonin can regulate our specific appetites: our cravings for carbohydrates or protein.[39,40] Diets high in carbohydrates and low in protein impact the system by raising insulin levels and increasing the odds of L-tryptophan getting into the brain. When converted to serotonin it results in a decreased appetite for cookies, cake, ice cream, and all the basic ingredients of binge eating. The opposite is true if we eat a protein-rich diet. A protein-rich diet lowers serotonin levels and enhances the chances of carbohydrate binge eating. Diets made up largely of complex carbohydrates and less than 10 percent protein have been shown to reduce such binge eating in both animals and obese people who have histories of occasionally putting down a gallon of Rocky Road ice cream or a couple of pounds of chocolate chip cookies. This ancient specific appetite program most likely served to get us out of the caves now and then to supplement our carbohydrate diets with a little protein. Carbohydrates were easy to come by, but mice were hard to catch.

While carbohydrate intake can affect specific appetites and binge eating in rats, things are more complicated among humans, where specific appetites, binge eating, depression, and obesity appear to be interrelated. Carbohydrate craving and between-meal carbohydrate snacking, which elevates serotonin levels in our brains, might well be an attempt to change how we feel emotionally rather than a response to food deprivation. The Wurtmans suggest that at least 50 percent of the obese people who crave and snack on carbohydrates do so because of a biological need to elevate their moods. Obese carbohydrate-cravers invariably snack on carbohydrates even when protein snacks are available, and such snacking amounts to about one-third of their daily caloric intake. When given the drug D-fenfluramine (which increases serotonin levels in their brains), they cut down snacking by about 40 percent. Thus some of us may snack on carbohyrates to treat our depressions.

The serotonin precursor L-tryptophan has been successfully used to reduce depression in some people. Since L-tryptophan elevates brain serotonin levels, it is thought that depression may be associated with serotonin deficiency. Dr. Marie Åsberg[2] and others have hypothesized that "serotonin depression" may be a separate form of depression, a biochemical subgroup which exists within the larger family of affective disorders. One research group has suggested that profoundly low serotonin levels might be critical markers for predicting future suicide.[3] This extreme serotonin deficiency has been referred to as the *suicide factor* and has been the focus of considerable research.

A number of special groups of people are characterized by having below-average serotonin levels. Besides those who are depressed and potentially suicidal, they include alcoholics, chronic marijuana users, and sensation-seeking individuals who engage in

high-risk sports such as mountain climbing. It has been hypothesized that people who either attempt or successfully commit suicide, as well as those who climb mountains, act out their anxiety
instead of tolerating it or tranquilizing it with alcohol or marijuana.[11]

Serotonin contributes to our sex drive and also reduces our pain
sensitivity. In cultures where the natural food supply contains too
little L-tryptophan, men have fewer erections and are more sensitive
to pain. One powerful antidepressant drug (clomipramine) elevates
serotonin levels dramatically and shows great promise as a treatment for obsessive-compulsive disorders.

Just as dopamine levels seem to be linked to extraversion,
serotonin levels also appear to be tied to personality. Serotonin
levels are related to which of us lead and which of us follow. Male
primates (baboons as well as humans) who are in leadership positions have higher serotonin levels.

Norepinephrine

Norepinephrine is implicated in panic attacks, terrifying experiences which can develop into agoraphobia. Mild electrical
stimulation of the locus coeruleus, a brain-stem area rich in norepinephrine neurons, results in panic reactions in monkeys. Surgically damaging the area erases a capacity for such fearful behavior. Three classes of drugs (monoamine-oxidase-inhibiting and
tricyclic antidepressants and the benzodiazepine alprazolam)
which impact norepinephrine function have been shown to relieve
panic attacks. With such clear physiological correlates, it is not
surprising that panic disorders appear to have a genetic basis.

We are at highest risk if we have an identical twin (that is, with
the same genetic makeup) who suffers from the disorder. We are
also more vulnerable if we have relatives who have a history of
panic attacks. Women are more susceptible than men. Endo-
crinologist Dr. Daniel Carr suggests that progesterone, which is
secreted during the luteal phase of the menstrual cycle, may enhance the sensitivity of the chemoceptors which trigger anxiety.[10]

Depression has been also associated with a deficiency of norepinephrine. The antidepressant drug desipramine, which significantly elevates norepinephrine activity, activates and relieves de-

pression in individuals who suffer from a generalized slowing of physical and emotional reactions (psychomotor retardation). Some depressed patients have been successfully treated with large doses of tyrosine, a large dietary amino acid which is a precurser for norepinephrine.[39]

Serotonin and Norepinephrine

A review of the research concerning serotonin and nor-epinephrine deficiency concludes that, while the evidence is indirect, there is compelling evidence to support the hypothesis that two important subtypes of depression are associated with low brain turnover rates of these two neurotransmitters.[12] The reviewers point out (1) that the drugs which affect our central nervous system amines (serotonin and norepinephrine) alter our mood states; (2) that neuroendocrine studies suggest functional abnormalities in the central aminergic systems of those of us with mood disorders; and (3) that urinary and cerebrospinal-fluid amine-metabolite levels have been found to be altered among some depressed patients (when enzymes break down or degrade neurotransmitters the resulting substance is referred to as a *metabolite*). The reviewers argue that some of us suffer a form of depression which is characterized by a low turnover rate of brain serotonin, and that others suffer another form which reflects low nor-epinephrine activity in our brains.

Recent research which associates neurotransmitter deficiencies and suicide suggests that extreme norepinephrine deficiency may be as much of a warning sign for potential suicide as low levels of serotonin. This research is very intriguing because both impulsivity and aggression enter the picture.

Dr. Steven Secunda has discussed some of the relevant work.[27] He and his associates point out that violent suicide attempters have low levels of 5-HIAA (a serotonin metabolite found in the cerebrospinal fluid). They also point out that both high *and* low levels of MHPG (a norepinephrine metabolite found in the blood and the urine) are associated with increased suicidal symptoms among depressed patients. Thus those who attempt suicide appear to have below-average serotonin activity and either below- or above-average norepinephrine activity. Secunda found lower MHPG levels in their suicide attempter group than in the nonattempters, but no differences in 5-HIAA, suggesting that the critical variable for predicting suicide attempts might be norepinephrine inactivity.

The detective story continues with the discovery that individuals with a history of either suicide attempts *or* aggressive behavior *both* have low 5-HIAA levels (reflecting serotonin inactivity).[5] Then a third research group checked out 5-HIAA levels among violent criminals and found that the levels of this metabolite were lower among impulsive criminals than among those who committed premeditated violent acts.[18] Thus low serotonin activity might mark impulsive behavior.

Finally, a group headed up by Dr. John Mann conducted postmortem examinations on suicide victims and discovered evidence of reduced noradrenergic (norepinephrine) activity in their brains.[19] Mann points out that other laboratories have found that increased noradrenergic activity is related to aggression. He suggests that while reduced serotonergic activity might set off violent, impulsive acts, noradrenergic and dopaminergic systems might determine the direction of the violent impulsive act. Unusually high norepinephrine turnover would turn the violence outward in aggression, while abnormally low norepinephrine turnover would more likely result in the violence being turned inward, resulting in a suicide attempt.

Beta Endorphin

Beta endorphin is a neuromodulator which has received considerable notoriety because it is a chemical key which opens the same euphoric doors as opium or morphine. It also functions as a neuromodulator by regulating the release of Substance P, a neurotransmitter which modulates pain.

The pain-free and numbed-out shock state which follows severe injury is an example of these "endogenous" (internally produced) "opiates" (morphinelike substances) at work. They may play a role in the emotional euphoria called *runners high*, and are what allows injured athletes to continue to "play hurt." The pain relief which comes from acupuncture is mediated by beta endorphin, which is activated in response to having needles stuck into us. Beta endorphin also has a significant role in pregnancy and postpartum pain. During pregnancy, levels gradually rise and peak at as much as 10 times normal. The abrupt postdelivery drop in beta endorphin may contribute to the depression experienced by some women. Beta endorphin levels are also linked to sexual drive and behavior. Our sex drive is strongest during the "good times" when stress and related endorphin levels are low.

Perhaps of more significance is research which suggests that the opiate system may play a role in autism and in eating disorders. The drug naloxone, which blocks opiate activity, has been shown to reduce symptoms in some autistic children.[13] If opiates do play a role in autism, this role would provide a biological explanation for why these children seem relatively immune from pain, and why they have such low needs for social stimulation. It may also be possible that serotonin has a role in autism. About a third of the autistic children examined by one research team had an antibody which interfered with serotonergic activity.[32]

It has been hypothesized that opiates are involved in anorexia nervosa, since the opioid system reacts to immediate and prolonged food deprivation. Starvation results in opiate release and an initial feeling of euphoria in all of us. This makes evolutionary sense, if you think about more primitive times when periodic deprivation was not uncommon. It further makes sense that the opiate system would shut down when starvation became prolonged. Uncomfortable hunger pain would motivate us to start searching for food. At least this would be the case if our systems worked normally. One theory is that some people who suffer from anorexia nervosa do not have a functional opiate shut-down mechanism. Another line of thought is that the beta endorphin response to the stress produced by the self-induced vomiting of individuals who suffer from bulimia nervosa might somehow reinforce their cycles of fasting and binge-eating behavior. Bulimics and anorexics frequently have abnormal endorphin levels.

Even though most of us are neither bulimic nor anorectic, endorphins may contribute to our weight control problems in that they appear to cause certain foods to taste especially good. It has been discovered that rats who have been fully fed will begin to enthusiastically feed on fats, proteins, and sweets if injected with a small amount of beta endorphin.[13] This makes survival sense, in that these foods will satiate an animal longer than carbohydrates. Obese people, if given the opiate antagonist naloxone, will eat less.

Research on beta endorphin's possible role in both autism and the eating disorders has just begun and for the most part permits only speculation at this early stage. There is an absence of research and replication of early work. If beta endorphin turns out to play a role in even a small percentage of the individuals who suffer from these disorders, the drug naloxone, which blocks opiate activity, may turn out to be a viable intervention.

The opiates may also be a critical link between stress and physical disease. Opiates released during continuing stress are very likely implicated in both ulceration and atherosclerosis (the narrowing and hardening of arteries through cholesterol buildup on arterial walls). On the other hand, endorphins appear to bolster our immune system.

One study has suggested that physical contact with mothers stimulates opiate release in infant animals. Seems possible, since warmth alone can stimulate endorphin activity. If cuddling up with Mom has an effect similar to a small injection of heroin, it could explain why it is possible to kiss away minor hurts, why some of us seek a lot of physical contact with others, and why some of us get permanently hooked on our mothers. It remains for future research to convincingly determine whether or not opiate activity is involved in social bonding.

Acetylcholine

Acetylcholine has been under renewed scrutiny of late. Acetylcholine deficiency has long been associated with Alzheimer's disease, and now it appears that this neurotransmitter may also bear some relationship to depression, at least as a potential marker. We have known for decades that the most serious forms of depression tend to run in families, and now it has been discovered that those of us who suffer from, or have in the past suffered from, unipolar and bipolar depressive disorders, have an overabundance of acetylcholine receptor sites in skin cells.[22] This finding could lead to a test for vulnerability to bipolar and unipolar depressive disorders and early treatment intervention in children and adolescents.

These findings also relate to a hypothesis that relates to biogenic system imbalance and depression. One group of researchers suggests that depression is associated with increased cholinergic (acetylcholine) activity, and that mania is associated with increased noradrenergic (norepinephrine) activity.[14] Dr. Solomon Snyder points out that this hypothesis rests on the unproven assumption that the genetic factors which regulate cholinergic receptor density in peripheral cells such as the skin do the same in the brain. He suggests that there is experimental support for the hypothesis that depression may be rooted in excessive cholinergic activity in that the effectiveness of the tricyclic antidepressant drugs is directly related to their ability to block cholinergic receptors.[31]

Biochemistry and Behavior

Provocative as these neurochemical breakthroughs may be, they provide only an exciting new wedge into our understanding of mental disorders. In the world of mental disorders, cause and effect can become confused.

Genetically predisposed neurochemical system imbalances such as an overactive dopamine or acetylcholine system may influence our behavior, predisposing us to schizophrenia or depression. But on the other hand, prolonged stress and our learned ways of coping with stress (adaptive behaviors which minimize it, or maladaptive behaviors which exacerbate it) can also influence our neurochemical systems. A prolonged stress reaction, for example, can result in physiological consequences such as ulceration, atherosclerosis, or a depressed immune system. It can also result in a depletion of critical neuromodulators which can affect mood and behavior. Prolonged stress, for example, may overwhelm or deplete a neurotransmitter system which ordinarily inhibits anxiety and panic, as well as other systems where insufficiency results in depression. And what is worse is that the drugs which are prescribed to normalize behavior may also exacerbate the systemic imbalance which predisposed us to the original disorder. For example, continued use of antipsychotic medication which blocks dopamine receptor sites may result in a sensitization or proliferation of those sites. The interplay between genetic predisposition (inherited biological system imbalance), environment, personality, and behavior is a complex one. All of these factors interact and enter into the formula which determines the probability of developing a mental disorder.

Nonetheless, these early discoveries of genetic and biochemical bases of mental disorders are of significant value. They provide markers to identify those of us who are at risk of developing such disorders, and have facilitated the development of drugs to treat serious disorders which have been historically untreatable. They also allow us to make sensible decisions about how we live, since factors such as stress, diet, street drugs such as amphetamine, and exercise can all impact these systems which are so involved in several mental disorders.

Psychosocial Factors

Causes of our mental disorders cover a broad spectrum, all the way from an organic defect to the ways in which members of our family react to our behavior. For example, let's hypothesize that there is a biochemical predisposition, perhaps a shortage of a particular enzyme or some sort of systemic imbalance, which might render us vulnerable to alcohol addiction. Whether or not we ever become dependent upon alcohol depends on a vast number of factors. They would include how our personalities and self-concepts are shaped within our families and sociocultural environment, whether a stressor of sufficient intensity comes along to trigger and help maintain our drinking, and how our family members react to our dependency (whether they become enablers who somehow reinforce it and unknowingly make the problem worse).

We were not all created equal. Some of us suffer genetic and congenital defects. Others of us don't have our primary physical needs met or do not experience adequate environmental stimulation and activity. Even our physiques and the degree to which we meet our culture's definitions of what is attractive can influence our psychological development.

Those of us who were dealt an average or better genetic hand can be emotionally damaged by what we experience within our sociocultural environment and families. Those of us born into low socioeconomic status and in our inner cities have a tougher time. Society sometimes also demands that we assume roles, such as fighting in wars, which cause deep personal conflict. Some of us are the victims of prejudice, unemployment, or unpredictable social change.

It is in the psychosocial arena, largely within our families, that we unconsciously learn whether or not we are of worth, whether or not our needs are as important as those of others, and whether or not we are lovable. It is here that we learn whether or not the world is a safe and predictable place, a place which has room for our hopes. It is here where we learn independence and confidence in our ability to meet and deal with life's stresses—or learn helplessness, dependence, and games to manipulate or solicit caretaking from others. Roles, trust, sexuality, and the whole complex structure which we refer to as personality are largely formed in this arena.

Deprivation, abuse, and trauma all leave deep scars, and often the worst are inflicted at home by the people we most trust and on whom we must depend. In 1984 nearly 3 out of every 100 children in America were reported to child-protective agencies as being the victims of physical, sexual, or psychological abuse. We can only speculate on the number unreported, but one recent poll suggests that about one of every four to five adult Americans has been a victim of childhood sexual abuse.[36] Traumatic abusive experiences leave some of us so deeply scarred that we will never again feel trust in or compassion for others.

Some us are parented inadequately. Our parents may be overprotective or overly indulgent. They may be very inconsistent in disciplining us or may communicate with us in destructive irrational ways. Some parents model maladaptive and antisocial behaviors which will cause us trouble in the future.

All of us carry emotional scars, and we will all scar others no matter how well-meaning we are. Just as our parents were imperfect, we, too, will be imperfect parents. No one can protect us, nor can we protect our children from loss and pain. We must each, in our own way, learn how to deal with life's problems and the emotions which they engender. And when push comes to shove, when we are profoundly threatened and our backs are up against the wall, we each have our final redoubt. For some of us it is withdrawal and emotional numbness. Some of us automatically blame and attack. Others of us become helpless, irrational, or hysterical. Some drink. Whether our behavior is adaptive or maladaptive, we learn to do whatever works for us.

Thus, all of us have unconsciously learned how to somehow protect ourselves from the threats we encounter, and our personalities reflect these typical ways of dealing with other people. Some of us grow up to be reasonably trusting, responsible, independent adults who are capable of entering into and maintaining healthy, reciprocal interpersonal relationships. Others of us are not so lucky. Our learned patterns of behavior are maladaptive. Mental disorders which are unconsciously learned in interpersonal relationships are best unlearned in interpersonal relationships. Psychotherapy can provide a variety of structured social circumstances where such relearning can take place.

This book, however, is not largely concerned with the many mental disorders which have roots largely in experience and unconscious learning, the sorts of disorders which are the usual targets of psychotherapeutic treatments. Its primary focus is on how exercise might effectively treat symptomatic depression and anxiety. Therefore our interest in mental disorders which have psychogenic origins is largely restricted to the fact that many of these maladaptive behavior patterns both cause and perpetuate depression and anxiety.

With mental disorders resulting from the complex interplay of so many determiners, treatment can present a dilemma. Let's have a look now at biochemical and psychotherapeutic treatments.

Chapter 4
Biochemical Treatments

Twenty million Americans suffer from biologically determined mental disorders, and an equal number of us carry biological predispositions for various mental disorders.

The history of humankind includes a history of psychotic individuals who have been virtually untreatable. During the first half of this century our mental hospital populations grew larger and larger with each passing year. Largely custodial care was provided for chronically ill people who would present a danger to themselves or others if they remained uncared for. Many hallucinated and were delusional, out of touch with reality. Others could become unpredictably out of control and violent. Some were so depressed that they could not care for themselves and would eventually die if left alone. Many of these seriously ill people came from families where there was a history of schizophrenia or severe depression, but the extent to which the illnesses were genetically passed on was not known. Perhaps these disabling diseases were partially the result of living with parents and other family members who suffered from similar severe behavior disorders.

During the first half of this century mental hospitals were overcrowded, understaffed, and underfunded. There was little money for treatment or research, and with each passing year the number of patients in American mental hospitals increased. The major treatments during this period were restraint, chemical sedation, electroconvulsive therapy (ECT), and prefrontal lobotomy.

The lobotomy was a surgical procedure which rather haphazardly severed neural pathways in the brain. These pathways connected the brain areas for organized thought in the frontal cortex to those which regulated emotion around the hypothalamus. The use of lobotomies peaked in response to the influx of World War II veterans in the 1940s. The surgery did calm agitated patients and help reduce mental hospital overpopulations, but its side effects were serious and sometimes horrendous. It often quite simply dehumanized people. Both lobotomies and ECT were sometimes used on the wrong people and for the wrong reasons.

Then, around 1950 medical breakthroughs in France and Australia forever changed the lives of those who crowded our mental hospitals. Prefrontal lobotomies stopped, ECT was refined and selectively administered, and hundreds of thousands of patients, for better or for worse, left mental hospitals.

Chlorpromazine and Schizophrenia

In the early 1950s French scientists synthesized a substance called *chlorpromazine* for possible use as an antihistamine. While the drug proved to be far too sedative to be useful as an antihistamine, it caught the attention of two psychiatrists who decided to see whether it might work to calm down schizophrenic patients. They discovered that it had an almost unbelievable dual effect: quieting hyperactive patients and activating those who were withdrawn. It became the first of a family of antipsychotic drugs which, for the first time, did more than simply sedate patients. It had very specific antipsychotic functions, including the reduction of hallucinations, delusions, and thought disorders. This remarkable drug was soon in use all over the world, and it transformed the lives of those suffering from schizophrenia.

While the antipsychotic drugs have many serious side effects and don't actually cure schizophrenia, they have offered the first significant alternative to the out-of-control terror of psychotic episodes and the social isolation of a life on the back wards of our then burgeoning mental hospitals. For the first time many patients became accessible for social interventions and psychotherapy, therapy which might help them to avoid future psychotic episodes. Under the trade name Thorazine in this country, chlorpromazine closed many of our mental hospitals. After 50,000 years of *Homo sapiens sapiens* history, the first effective tool for reducing psychotic symptoms had been discovered. Chlorpromazine constituted a major medical breakthrough.[11]

Lithium and the Bipolar Mood Disorders

Meanwhile, in Australia, a physician was experimenting with the drug lithium carbonate in an attempt to reduce sodium retention in cardiac patients. He serendipitously discovered that it was highly effective in normalizing manic patients who suffered from bipolar mood disorders. Because large doses were lethal, and because no one yet knew what constituted a normal range, American physicians adopted a hands-off posture until Danish researchers established the drug's effectiveness and safe administration. Lithium may be the most astounding drug ever discovered for the treatment of mental disorders. Used prophylactically it can prevent recurrent manic and depressive states, and it can normalize those suffering manic states—people who in the past could only be sedated and restrained. Thanks to the Australian Dr. John Cade, those of us who inherited genetic defects which would ordinarily predispose us to a lifetime with a disabling bipolar mood disorder can live more reasonably normal lives. Lithium is the treatment of choice for bipolar disorders. To date, nothing else has worked better.[11]

Recent research has indicated that lithium is also effective for some (but not all) individuals who suffer from unipolar depression (major depression). This suggests that depressions might actually be families of disorders made up of subclasses with different causes. Dr. David Jimerson has reviewed recent studies concerning the role of dopamine in depression.[4] He points out that functional dopamine activity is reduced in some subgroups of depressed patients and is increased in manic patients. Jimerson concludes that many investigations now suggest that both the antidepressant drugs and lithium have important regulatory effects on forebrain postsynaptic dopamine receptors.

Lithium also has some side effects. It can cause lethargy, affect our motor coordination, and cause some gastrointestinal problems. As with many other drugs, very long-term use can cause kidney malfunction or even damage.

Electroconvulsive Therapy

ECT was dramatized by novelist Ken Kesey in *One Flew over the Cuckoo's Nest*. The hero, a lovable and moderately psychopathic character, didn't even belong in a mental hospital but was eventually given ECT as punishment for challenging the system. A colleague of mine who was a psychologist on the ward where Kesey worked as a technician while writing his book reassured me that Kesey's work of fiction is just that. Nonetheless, Kesey let it be known that ECT was sometimes inappropriately used and abused even after it was quite apparent that its effectiveness was largely limited to relieving the symptoms of major depression. Its controversial nature was reflected in an ordinance which forbid its use in Berkeley, California, for a number of years.

ECT may forever remain the center of controversy, since the notion of delivering a seizure-producing electric shock to someone's brain is difficult for most of us to accept. However, responsible researchers remain at odds concerning the seriousness and permanence of the side effects of the procedure. Patients report disorientation, confusion, memory loss, and impaired capacity for learning following ECT. The first two side effects are clearly short-term. The controversy concerns amnesia or memory loss.

Memory loss has been reduced by replacing sine-wave with brief-pulse-wave electrical current and by administering it to only the nondominant brain hemisphere. But the debate continues and centers on whether the memory loss effects are short-term or permanent. Some who receive ECT appear to suffer both serious and permanent memory loss, being forced to retire from employment with permanent disability. Others have little or no impairment. During 1987, 2614 patients received ECT in California. Of those, 627, or about 1 in 4, complained of memory problems.[10]

Patients are given a general anesthesia and a muscle relaxant prior to being given ECT, and while only a small fraction of the electrical current applied to the skin on a patient's skull reaches the brain, it must be sufficient to produce a brain seizure if it is to be effective. It doesn't take much. Electricity sufficient to make a 100-watt light bulb flicker causes frantic neural activity in our brains.[10]

The effect of ECT is complex. It alters almost every aspect of brain activity. One theory is that it may be the brain's reaction to the seizure which produces a reduction in depression. The brain reacts to the seizure by producing higher levels of an amino acid neurotransmitter called *GABA* (gamma aminobutyric acid), which sharply inhibits activity in cortical areas which appear to be overactive in depressed patients. Studies show that ECT has an acute (immediate) effect that is precisely duplicated over the course of about three weeks by the clinically effective antidepressant drugs. Both ECT and antidepressant drugs reduce the sensitivity of a particular system in the brain (the norepinephrine-coupled adenylate cyclase system in the limbic forebrain and frontal cortex).[5,6]

Why then, if the effects of ECT can at least in part be duplicated by antidepressant drugs, is it reemerging as an increasingly accepted medical tool? The answer is that it acts so very rapidly and is so highly effective. It is the only effective treatment for those deeply depressed people who have not responded to either biochemical or psychotherapeutic treatment, people who would likely die from self-neglect if left to their own devices. It is often the treatment of last resort.[2]

About 70 to 80 percent of patients who receive four to six ECT treatments show complete remission of symptoms, a far higher success rate than the 50 to 60 percent seen when unipolar depressed patients are treated with antidepressant drugs or psychotherapy. But like the antipsychotic drugs, ECT is not a cure, and its effects may not be permanent. One series of treatments is not always enough. However, it can terminate immobilizing and life-threatening deep depression and can be followed up with maintenance antidepressant-drug therapy and psychotherapy.

Far from being a primitive device used to punish and control disadvantaged patients in public institutions, ECT is now used largely in university and private hospitals to treat middle- and upper-income women. In California, where precise records on ECT are maintained, women patients outnumber men by two to one, and about half of them are over the age of 65.[10] Between 60,000 and 100,000 patients receive ECT each year in this country, and many patients feel that ECT treatment is less traumatic than a visit to the dentist.[9] Most patients require 6 to 12 treatments over the course of two to four weeks. Treatments currently cost $800 to $1000 dollars each, and can be administered on an outpatient basis. When contrasted to a long inpatient stay in a hospital which carries no guarantee that symptoms will abate, ECT is a very cost-effective treatment, and it is as safe as any procedure where a general anesthetic is involved. The side effects remain a serious concern, but for many patients they are an acceptable trade-off for ending an incapacitating depression which will not respond to any other form of treatment.

A recent National Institute of Mental Health panel of experts consisting of psychiatrists, psychologists, and lawyers issued a position statement indicating that ECT is a safe and effective therapy for a narrow group of very serious mental illnesses (depression, mania, and schizophrenia) that more research should be done on ECT, and that ECT administration should be included in the training of future psychiatrists.[7]

The Antidepressant Drugs and Unipolar Depression

As in the case of lithium and chlorpromazine, the first effective antidepressant drug was discovered quite by accident when the antituberculosis drug isoniazid was found to elevate mood in depressed patients. The first of a group of antidepressants called *monoamine oxidase inhibitors* (MAOIs) was a close relative called iproniazid.

Monoamine oxidase (MAO) is an enzyme which breaks down or metabolizes various amines, including the mood-relevant neuromodulators dopamine, norepinephrine, and serotonin. Since unipolar depression has been associated with deficiencies and inactivity in both serotonergic and norepinephrine systems, one way to increase the number of these critical neuromodulators in synapses is to inhibit the action of MAO. The MAOIs accomplish just that, and they do reduce depression, but they have potentially dangerous and possibly lethal side effects.

The problem with the MAOIs is that monoamine oxidase not only breaks down the amines which are concerned with neural transmission, but also breaks down all amines, including other dietary amines which have critical roles in our well-being. Tyramine, for example, is found in common foods such as beer, wine, cheese, and liver. If tyramine builds up in our systems it can produce a dangerous and potentially fatal hypertensive condition. Those of us taking MAOIs must be very careful about our drinking and our diets. For this reason the MAOIs are prescribed only if patients fail to respond to other antidepressant medications. Why these drugs sometimes work when others fail is not clear at this juncture. Common MAOIs are Nardil, Parnate, and Marplan.

The most widely prescribed antidepressant drugs are the *tricyclic antidepressants* (TADs), so named because of their three-ring molecular structure. At least a part of their action, like that of the MAOIs, occurs at synapses. While the MAOIs inhibit the breakdown of amine neurotransmitters such as dopamine, serotonin, and norepinephrine, the TADs function by blocking their reuptake back into the presynaptic neuron where they are stored for future use. This blocking mechanism keeps more neurotransmitters within the synapse (available to bind on postsynaptic receptor sites), perhaps enough to activate a sluggish system. Various TADs are selective in blocking the reuptake of different neurotransmitters. Fluoxetine, for example, selectively blocks serotonin reuptake and has a negligible effect on norepinephrine. Imipramine (Tofranil) and amitriptyline (Elavil) also block serotonin reuptake (which has a sedating effect), but their first metabolites function to block norepinephrine uptake, and this "cascading metabolite effect" might largely account for the fact that these serotonergic drugs have an antidepressant effect. Desipramine (the first metabolite of imipramine) selectively blocks the reuptake of norepinephrine, and is prescribed as a highly activating antidepressant for individuals who are lethargic.

The fact that TADs function to block neurotransmitter reuptake within hours, but that their antidepressant effects aren't realized for about three weeks, suggests that significant postsynaptic events figure heavily in their antidepressant effects. Studies suggest that the suppression of a norepinephrine-coupled system in the limbic forebrain is the critical event.[5,6] The only antidepressants which effectively suppress this system are those which elevate norepinephrine activity. Drugs which activate only serotonergic systems won't do the job. ECT has precisely the same effect on this limbic forebrain system, but it accomplishes it immediately, while the antidepressants require several weeks to do the job. Even tyrosine, a dietary norepinephrine precursor, has been shown to effectively reduce depression in some individuals. All of the clinically effective TADs also block receptors for the neurotransmitter histamine, while the MAOIs do not.

The TADS, like nearly all drugs, have unpleasant side effects. Perhaps the most commonly complained about are their sedating effects and their contribution to weight gain. They also have hypertensive effects and affect cardiac action. They also lower seizure thresholds. Because of these and many other potential problems, the dosage for depressed individuals is very cautiously increased over the course of several weeks. If TADs don't work, MAOIs may be effective. Antidepressants cannot be taken forever. As the patient's systems adapt to the drug, an increased dosage or a switch to a new form of antidepressant may be required.

Antidepressants and Panic Disorder

Both TADs and MAOIs have been successfully used with some patients to reduce the frequency of panic attacks. A recent award-winning investigation done by Dr. Dennis Charney and his colleagues at the Yale University School of Medicine provides up-to-date information on this topic.[1] They compared the effectiveness of three antidepressant drugs in a group of patients who suffered from panic attacks (either with or without agoraphobia). One of the drugs was the tricyclic antidepressant imipramine, which has primary serotonergic and secondary norepinephrine functions, which we have outlined earlier. The other two drugs were from a new family (second generation) of antidepressants, triazolobenzodiazepine (alprazolam or Xanax) which also has anti-anxiety properties, and triazolopyridine (Trazodone), which strongly enhances serotonergic activity but has an insignificant impact on norepinephrine activity.

The results of this experiment were consistent with earlier related work. The researchers found that both imipramine and alprazolam were very effective in reducing the symptoms of general anxiety, the frequency of panic attacks, and phobic avoidance. The difference was that alprazolam was effective within the first week of treatment, while the effects of imipramine were not clinically apparent until the third or fourth week of treatment. Trazodone, which affects only serotonin activity, was ineffective.

This research suggests that panic attacks can be effectively treated with drugs which alter norepinephrine function in the brain, and that the two effective drugs probably alter these functions via different mechanisms. Alprazolam, which changes the shape of the receptor sites it occupies, may interact with GABA metabolism to lessen anxiety.[3] The researchers recommend that patients who suffer from panic disorder should be started off on a combination of alprazolam and imipramine for four to six weeks. By then, imipramine should control the symptoms and the patient can discontinue the alprazolam (which has dependency-producing properties).

Clomipramine and Obsessive-Compulsive Disorders

There is another TAD which differs from imipramine by only a single chlorine atom, but which has an even stronger effect in elevating serotonin levels. Developed in France in 1965, it is called clomipramine (Anafranil) and is widely used outside of the United States. It is now being tested for approval in this country because of its powerful and highly specific effect on obsessive-compulsive disorders (OCDs). Anafranil is reported to reduce symptoms dramatically in 15 percent and substantially in an additional 65 percent of patients suffering from OCDs. Some can resume normal life with such drug treatment alone, while for others the drug controls symptoms sufficiently to allow them to benefit from behavior therapy. More than a half-dozen studies have now demonstrated that clomipramine reduces OCD symptoms more effectively than any other drug, and suggest that such disorders might have a basis in serotonin deficiency.[8]

The problem is that while clomipramine's primary effect is to block the reuptake of serotonin, the secondary effect of one of its metabolites is to block reuptake of norepinephrine. To get to the bottom of things, Dr. Teri Perse[8] of the University of Wisconsin tested the effectiveness of fluvoxamine, an even more effective serotonin reuptake blocker which has no effect on norepinephrine function. Perse found fluvoxamine to be a highly effective drug for the treatment of obsessive-compulsive disorders, and the study has since been replicated with similar results. It appears that obsessive-compulsive disorders are rooted in or at least associated with serotonergic-system deficiency.

Perse, whose treatment review concerning obsessive-compulsive disorders won an award, suggests that compulsive patients, those who ritualistically act out repeated behavior sequences, be first treated with behavior psychotherapy techniques. These techniques are effective about 70 to 80 percent of the time. Perse cites studies which suggest that behavior therapy techniques have not reduced obsessive symptoms (uncontrolled ruminations) as effectively as they have compulsive symptoms. For those compulsive patients who do not respond to behavior therapy, Perse suggests biochemical treatment with clomipramine or fluvoxamine, which have been shown to be effective in about 80 percent of cases. For those few patients who fail to respond to either treatment, Perse points out that psychosurgery is a viable option and that stereotactic limbic leucotomy has been shown to be safe and effective. This operation involves making two small lesions in the lower medial quadrant of the frontal lobe. The lesions course through the cingulate gyrus and interrupt frontolimbic connections.

The Benzodiazepines, Anxiety, and Phobias

The minor tranquilizers are a mixed blessing. The earliest one, meprobamate, appeared to function largely through muscle relaxation and was marketed as Miltown or Equanil. The meprobamates were quickly replaced by a rapidly multiplying family of benzodiazepines such as Librium, Valium, Dalmane, and more recently, Xanax. During the 1960s and 1970s the benzodiazepines were widely abused, both on the street and through legal prescriptions. Librium was America's most widely prescribed drug at one point. When the addictive properties of these drugs became apparent, limits were set on prescription procedures, but benzodiazepines are still widely used. In addition to being addictive, these minor tranquilizers can be lethal, especially when combined with alcohol. They also have metabolites which remain in our systems, resulting in the buildup of toxins. Dalmane, if taken for sleep each night, leaves toxins which may reach a critical level in as little as a week. All of these drugs cause drowsiness and lethargy, leaving us groggy and not fully functional in the morning. What's more, anxiety should never be thoughtlessly tranquilized away, since it often provides the motivation to face up to important issues and make necessary changes in our lives.

One of the reasons the benzodiazepines are so frequently abused is that they produce such marvelous tranquility. They have sedative, muscle-relaxing, and anxiety-reducing qualities. But their most remarkable quality is their capacity to selectively reduce fear or anxiety while leaving adaptive behaviors intact. Thus, they have application in the treatment of phobias and generalized anxiety disorders. Both Xanax and the antidepressant imipramine have been shown to effectively reduce phobic avoidance responses. Xanax, while faster acting, is a poor choice since it can produce dependency.

Conclusions

Biochemical interventions are the treatments of choice to relieve the symptoms of those very severe mental disorders which are genetically predisposed and are products of biochemical deficiencies and imbalances, disorders whose symptoms frequently appear to be independent of both experience and precipitating events. Schizophrenia, bipolar mood disorders, and some unipolar mood disorders fall into this group. Panic disorders, though less severe than the others, also qualify. These biochemical interventions do not "cure" these disorders, but they appear to be the only effective means of reducing the symptoms. This does not imply that psychotherapy is without a role in the treatment of some of these disorders, only that by itself, it is largely ineffective.

There is a second rough category of disorders where biological predisposition, environmental factors, and learned personality variables more obviously interact. These disorders often respond to either biochemical or psychotherapeutic interventions, or to combinations of the two. They include the various phobias, some depressions, obsessive-compulsive disorders, and substance abuse disorders. Where there is a choice, psychotherapy should be tried before resorting to psychoactive drugs (which all have moderate to dangerous side effects). Symptoms of depression and anxiety should not be arbitrarily taken away with medication, as they frequently are the consequence of maladaptive behavior patterns which should be attended to with psychotherapy. Simply reducing the symptoms of depression and anxiety with drugs may reduce the motivation to change the behavior patterns which cause us to be depressed or anxious.

Finally there is a category of disorders which have biochemical components, but are almost totally the result of social learning rather than predisposition and are most effectively treated with psychotherapies. Personality disorders and adjustment disorders, for example, make up a sizable share of the individuals who are treated by psychotherapists. Such disorders are of relevance to this book largely to the degree to which they result in anxiety and depression.

Summing Up

The current status of biochemical therapy for mental disorders looks something like this:

1. Pharmacologists have frequently led the way in developing theories of mental disorders by dramatizing the relationships between such disorders and biochemical-system imbalance.
2. The major breakthroughs in the treatment of mental disorders have been biochemical. Lithium and antipsychotic drugs such as chlorpromazine constitute medical landmarks. They are the only effective treatments for reducing the symptoms of bipolar disorders and schizophrenia.
3. Electroconvulsive therapy, controversial because of its side effects, is the most effective treatment for profound and disabling depression which has failed to respond to other interventions.
4. The antidepressant drugs are effective in reducing the symptoms of moderate and major depression in 50 to 60 percent of cases. The antidepressant clomipramine is highly effective in the treatment of obsessive-compulsive disor-

ders, and the antidepressant imipramine effectively reduces the occurrence of panic attacks.

5. The minor tranquilizers are useful to relieve symptomatic anxiety, to reduce phobic avoidance, to induce sleep, and to ease alcohol withdrawal. Xanax quickly reduces the frequency of panic attacks. These drugs are frequently abused.

6. All drugs have side effects which range from minor to very serious. Some are addictive. Some can be lethal. Because of side effects, biochemical treatments should not be prescribed if there is an effective alternative form of treatment available.

7. Drugs should not be arbitrarily prescribed to reduce symptoms which signal the need for psychotherapy.

While biochemical treatments are the only interventions which effectively treat some individuals, and combined biochemical and psychotherapeutic treatments are necessary for others, many of us suffer from mental disorders for which psychotherapy is the only effective treatment. Because so many individuals have learned maladaptive behavior patterns which, when repeatedly acted out, result in anxiety and depression, it is important that we now examine the effectiveness of psychotherapeutic treatments.

Chapter 5
The Psychotherapies

There was little hope for those who suffered from many mental disorders until around the turn of this century, when Freud developed the first theory and treatment techniques. Treatment remained in the hands of the medical profession until around the end of World War II. Psychiatrists were few, and their only psychotherapeutic tool was long-term psychoanalysis. Then, in the 1940s, tens of thousands of emotionally damaged war veterans came pouring back into the United States. Psychologists, who had been mainly doing research and diagnostic testing, and social workers, who had primarily interfaced with patient families, were drawn into the treatment arena.

With the help of the GI Bill, clinical psychology began to swell with new psychotherapists. During the postwar years they were busy developing new theories and techniques, treating patients, and teaching others how to treat patients. Unfortunately, there was no evidence that either psychoanalysis or any of the new forms of psychotherapy actually worked.

Does Psychotherapy Work?

It was in 1950 that the distinguished psychologist Dr. Vic Raimy, who was dismayed by the state of affairs, critically defined psychotherapy as, "An unidentified technique applied to unspecified problems with unpredictable outcomes."[14]

But it was not until 1952 that the eminent British psychologist Dr. Hans Eysenck caught everyone's attention. Eysenck had reviewed two dozen psychotherapy outcome studies which involved more than 7000 patients. He published a critical article which pointed out that most of the research which had been done was of poor quality and had proven nothing. Eysenck concluded that in the studies which he had reviewed, about two-thirds of neurotics spontaneously recovered on their own without any treatment whatsoever (over the course of two years), and that those few studies which had had adequate control groups showed that neurotics who were treated recovered at the same rates as those who were not treated. His conclusion was that psychotherapy made no difference in recovery rates.[4]

A few years later the respected psychologist Dr. Paul Meehl wondered how psychologists could continue to practice psychotherapy when it had not yet been proven to be effective. He pointed out that people spontaneously improve without psychotherapy and suggested that this same spontaneous remission of symptoms also occurred while people were in treatment, perpetuating the belief that the treatment had actually helped.[11]

Clinical psychologists, who were struggling for respectability as legitimate mental-health providers, were brought up short by all of this, especially by Eysenck's documented criticism. Faced with the fact that there was almost no respectable research proving the efficacy of psychotherapy, researchers began to design studies which would determine whether psychotherapy was better than no treatment at all.

Now, nearly 40 years later, it turns out that we can say with some confidence that psychotherapy is better than nothing. Just exactly how much better is not entirely clear, but it has been demonstrated to be at least moderately helpful.

Certainly one of the most significant things which has been discovered as a result of this large research effort on the effects of psychotherapy is that Eysenck was correct in pointing out that a substantial number of people suffering from mental disorders do, in fact, spontaneously recover without either drugs or psychotherapy. That many of us become symptom-free without having to invest time and money in treatment is very good news. Eysenck's early estimate that two out of three neurotics spontaneously recover over the course of two years is now generally considered high. In 1978, a major review of the available quality psychotherapy-outcome studies concluded that an average of about 43 percent of untreated people show symptom reduction and improvement.[2] The studies reviewed typically involved about four months of psychotherapeutic treatment, so the spontaneous recovery percentage should be viewed within that time frame. The reviewers also pointed out that some people get worse during psychotherapy but were unwilling to estimate deterioration rates. Their opinion, after evaluating the best of the relevant research concerning the efficacy of psychotherapy, was that it had a "modest positive effect."

In 1977, Drs. Mary Smith and Gene Glass did a meta-analysis of 375 psychotherapy-outcome studies.[18] They averaged the "effect sizes" of treatment and non-treatment and concluded that at the time treatment ended, the average patient who had received psychotherapy was better off than 75 percent of those who had not. While this suggests that psychotherapy is a very legitimate enterprise, a more careful look at the results reveals that there is a great deal of overlap in the amount of improvement shown by treated and untreated patients. It turns out that 75 percent of untreated patients fell within the range of improvement shown by treated patients at the time treatment terminated. Nonetheless, the findings were hailed as the first solid proof that psychotherapy was, in fact, better than no treatment.

This controversial meta-analysis was criticized on many legitimate grounds by responsible researchers. Eysenck referred to it as "mega-silliness," but Smith and Glass retorted that however imperfect some of the studies included in their analysis might have been, all of the studies revealed a small, but significant, benefit from psychotherapy.

A second, more refined meta-analysis of 143 more carefully selected high-quality studies by Drs. David and Diana Shapiro in 1982 was even more optimistic, suggesting that when psychotherapy ended, the average patient who had received psychotherapy was better off than 84 percent of untreated patients.[16] Once again it should be pointed out that a substantial percentage of the untreated patients (about 65 percent) fell within the range of improvement shown by the treated patients when treatment ended. But whether we view the psychotherapy glass as being half full or half empty, it is now clear that psychotherapy is somewhat better than no treatment.

Are Some Kinds of Psychotherapy Better Than Others?

At this juncture, research concerning the effectiveness of the various forms of psychotherapy suggests that it doesn't appear to make any difference what kind we choose. This issue has not been without controversy.

Smith and Glass addressed this issue in 1977 with a second meta-analysis of 374 outcome studies which they had previously analyzed. They concluded that

> Despite volumes devoted to the theoretical differences among different schools of psychotherapy, the results of research demonstrate negligible differences in the effects produced by different therapy types.

However, the Smith and Glass data were later reanalyzed in a somewhat different manner by another scientist, who found the brief cognitive and behavior therapies to be somewhat more effective than the long-term analytic and humanistic interpersonal varieties,[5] and the Shapiros, who did the second meta-analysis of a more select group of psychotherapy outcome studies, came to a similar conclusion.[17]

Researchers with a behavior therapy orientation contend that there are treatments of choice (that certain specific forms of treatments are more effective than others for specific disorders) and that the behavior therapies are most effective in the treatment of the phobic and compulsive anxiety disorders. The treatment of choice for phobias is a technique called *in vivo flooding* which involves the therapist leaving the office and accompanying the patient to the feared object or circumstance. The patient is forced to experience the anxiety which he or she has learned to avoid through phobic avoidance behaviors, and with repeated exposures to the feared stimulus in the safe hands of the therapist the anxiety response is extinguished.

In the case of compulsive disorders, exposure in vivo forces the patient to make contact with the feared object (e.g., public door handles which the patient fears are covered with dirt and germs) and then prevents the ritualistic behavior (hand washing). These sorts of treatments typically result in 70 to 80 percent of patients showing significant improvement, and follow-ups suggest that the effects are lasting.[13]

Similarly, the brief depression-specific cognitive-behavioral therapy developed by Dr. Aaron Beck and his associates has an outstanding record.[1] Beck reports several studies which show it to be as effective as the most effective antidepressant drug therapy, and further suggests that its effects are longer-lasting. The technique has also been adapted to the treatment of phobias and anxiety disorders.

Beck's theoretical concepts suggest that our depressions result from irrational ideas about ourselves, the world in which we live, and the future. These irrational ideas result in self-defeating and self-fulfilling maladaptive behaviors. Beck asks his patients to test out their illogical thinking in experiments in their social world, experiments where the suggested new behavior can break up old self-feeding thought and behavior patterns.

A second brief depression-specific therapy which, like Beck's approach, deals with here-and-now problems rather than historical determinants, is the brief interpersonal therapy developed by Dr. G. L. Klerman and associates.[8] Interpersonal therapy is designed to help patients recognize and modify maladaptive interpersonal behavior patterns which have perpetuated their depression. Klerman's system has not been evaluated as extensively as Beck's, but it appears to be quite effective.

The effectiveness of these two brief depression-specific therapies was recently tested against a widely used antidepressant drug (imipramine) in what has been described as a landmark investigation funded by the NIMH. The study took place in a number of community clinics across the country, where experienced therapists were given special training in either the Beck or the Klerman system. Depressed outpatients were then assigned to one of four groups. Those assigned to the control group received only a placebo (a chemically inert pill) and clinical management (periodic check-in and assessment) over the course of the 16-week experiment. Those assigned to the three treatment groups received brief cognitive-behavior therapy, brief interpersonal therapy, or treatment with the tricyclic antidepressant drug imipramine.

The results have not been fully reported, but substantial data are available.[22] About 30 percent of the patients who were in the placebo group showed improvement over the course of 16 weeks. However, between 50 and 60 percent of those in the three different kinds of treatment groups showed improvement over the same time period. Improvement was more rapid in the drug group, but by Week 12, the patients in all three treatment groups had improved equally. Surprisingly, whether treated with psychotherapy or drugs, the people in all three groups showed similar work and social adjustment at the time that the treatment ended. This experiment received a great deal of press, with headlines which proclaimed that psychotherapy had been proven to be as effective as drugs in the treatment of some forms of depression.

Behavior therapy has many forms and has been applied in a variety of ways to modify undesirable behavior. Aversive therapy, in which mild electric shocks are associated with the sight, smell, and taste of alcohol, was shown to be effective in controlling drinking way back in 1930.[23] Aversion therapy has been used successfully in conjunction with other therapies for alcoholic treatment up until recently, but it has come into disfavor because of obvious ethical concerns, and because other behavior techniques have proven to work as well. This sort of aversive treatment has been used to treat smoking, drug dependence, gambling, and even head-banging behavior in autistic children.

Another class of behavior therapies center on the shaping of behavior through positive reinforcement. These therapies are widely and successfully used in institutional settings to shape the behavior of chronic schizophrenic patients, retarded children, autistic children, and other disturbed children whose behavior has been out of control.

There is no consensus, however, that behavior therapy is more effective than other forms, even when it is applied to specific disorders for which it is reputed to be the treatment of choice. Reviewers have pointed out that the majority of investigations which suggest the superiority of behavior therapy have been laboratory analogues involving student volunteers with minor problems. A review of 13 studies which compared the systematic desensitization technique of behavior therapy with other therapy techniques in the treatment of phobias revealed that in only two cases was the behavior therapy superior, and that in one of those cases the superiority of behavior therapy over analytic therapy had disappeared by six-month follow-up.[19]

In 1986 the American Psychological Association devoted an entire special issue of *American Psychologist* to evaluating research on various aspects of psychotherapy. A large number of expert clinical psychologists who reviewed the full spectrum of psychotherapy outcome research in an article in that special issue concurred that at this early juncture no therapy is demonstrably better than any other.[19] They state,

> On balance, studies of better than average quality using patient populations show little advantage of behavioral over nonbehavioral methods in the treatment of affective and anxiety disorders.

These findings are unsettling, especially when one considers the vast diversity of both the theories and the techniques which face the bewildered consumer. However unsettling, these findings do provide a protective net for the unsophisticated, since any of the current 450 forms of psychotherapy appear to help about as much as the next.

Common Nonspecific Psychotherapeutic Factors

How can it be that such a diverse family of systems and treatments appears to yield such equivalent therapeutic effects?

One possibility is that different approaches actually do result in somewhat different therapeutic effects, but that such differences have been blurred by research constraints and lost in the statistical maze of meta-analyses. Future research may well show that there are clear treatments of choice, specific techniques which more effectively reduce symptoms of specific disorders.

Another possibility is that all therapies, from classical psychoanalysis to strategic family therapy, share some common nonspecific elements which are largely responsible for the therapeutic effects.

Common Therapist Factors

For example, effective therapists from *all disciplines* may be warm, understanding individuals who are able to focus reasonably objectively on patients and share an ability to move patients toward new ways of looking at things.

Dr. Hans Strupp, who recently was honored with a Distinguished Contribution Award by the American Psychological Association, headed up a research team at Vanderbilt University which produced what may well be the single best piece of research ever done on the outcome of psychotherapy.[20] Strupp's group demonstrated that common therapist characteristics may be an important nonspecific factor in psychotherapy.

Patients with a common matched diagnosis (withdrawn, agitated, depressed males) were carefully selected and randomly assigned to one of three groups. Some were seen by highly trained clinical psychologists, analytical and interpersonal psychotherapists who had an average of 23 years of experience. Patients in the second group were seen for a similar time period by "counselors," who, as was unknown by the students, were college professors from a variety of academic disciplines, faculty members who had reputations as being "good listeners," but who had received no formal training as psychotherapists. A third group of patients was put on hold (a waiting list) for the same time period.

The patients who received treatment improved slightly more than those who were untreated and kept on a waiting list. However, it made no difference whether those in the two treatment groups saw highly experienced professional psychologists or were seen by selected historians, mathematicians, or philosophers. Not all college professors are good listeners, but perhaps effective therapists share such a trait, irrespective of the form of psychotherapy practiced.

Common Patient Factors

Patients may also have some common characteristics. Regardless of the kind of therapy they happen upon, they typically self-disclose, experience strong emotions, and explore those feelings. Patients also come to therapy with an expectation that it will help, and they usually build some sort of positive alliance with their therapist. Patients almost always experience increased self-acceptance and self-efficacy. All of these things could contribute to therapeutic gains, regardless of the kind of therapy.

Common Processes

It is also possible that all therapies share some processes, or that a similar sequence of critical events occurs when therapy is successful. Family therapy authority Jay Haley has argued that all forms of therapy incorporate common treatment-effective paradoxical features and methods of dealing with patient resistance which might account for a substantial portion of the symptom reduction, even if the therapist may be unaware of them and how they contribute to therapeutic change.

Paradox and Resistance. Haley points out that the human relationship between therapist and patient is an unusually paradoxical one.[6] It is a kind of purchased intimacy where the focus and disclosure are almost exclusively unidirectional. It's a relationship where the one who exposes is expected to trust the one who does not, a form of intimacy which is contrary to real life.

What's more, most therapists who engage in long-term analytic or interpersonal therapy paradoxically maintain control over the therapeutic relationship. They "give" patients the responsibility of determining whatever happens or does not happen in the course of treatment. Thus, the patient determines not only what gets talked about, but also the speed and depth of uncovering difficult material. However, "giving" the patient control allows the therapist to remain in control of the relationship. If the patient wastes time, resists, actively hates the therapist, or regresses, the skillful therapist, like the master hypnotist, interprets or reframes the patient's behavior as a good sign that therapy is progressing nicely. The typical self-defeating tactics which the patient so successfully employs in controlling outside relationships with intimates don't work with a skilled therapist.

It is precisely because of this paradoxical control-tactic that the therapist has so much more to offer than others with whom the patient is involved in daily life. No matter how skillful the patient is at controlling other important people with his or her symptomatic games, those games won't work with the therapist. The patient must try alternative ways of behaving with the therapist, either taking responsibility for his or her behavior and change or quitting treatment.

Haley points out that many therapies, both long- and short-term, also consist of a kind of paradoxical *benevolent ordeal* which may account for a large part of patient change. In many kinds of psychotherapy the warm and understanding therapist benevolently agrees that the patient "cannot help" acting out his or her involuntary symptomatic behavior. The therapist also agrees that the symptom is not the client's fault. The patient was perhaps the victim of an unfortunate trauma or imperfect parenting. Finally, the therapist studiously avoids encouraging the patient to stop the symptomatic behavior. It's fruitless to tell someone to voluntarily stop doing something which she or he cannot help doing. Thus, the patient, who comes to a high-priced expert, seeking help and direction, is told that he or she is in charge of what happens or does not happen. What's more, the patient who comes seeking to change is not encouraged to change or to stop behaving symptomatically. In addition, depending on the kind of therapy, patients will be expected to expose their personal inadequacies and areas of sensitivity, and also to deal with anxiety-arousing and guilt-provoking material.

The therapist's role is a puzzling and paradoxical one. If the therapist were simply benevolent the patient could handle the relationship. If the therapist were an individual who did nothing but provide punishment the patient could seek out someone else. But the benevolent therapist provides a continuing ordeal which will continue for as long as the patient remains unchanged, clinging to old ways of conceptualizing and dealing with his or her problems. When the patient does change, both therapist and patient are likely to attribute the change to whatever principles and techniques are central to the therapy. They may attribute the change to the development of a trusting relationship, cognitive restructuring, insight, or interpretations. While many of these factors may play a role, the benevolent ordeal is always at work.

The Power of the Placebo

People have been aware of the placebo effect for thousands of years, but it gained a certain amount of respectability around the turn of the century when the preeminent British physician Sir William Osler suggested to his medical school students that they should consider most drugs and treatments essentially useless, and that the history of medicine was largely the history of the placebo effect.[12] A review of the research on the placebo effect reveals that placebo treatment has a significant effect in nearly all aspects of medicine.[15]

Dr. Sean O'Connell has written an excellent article which spells out how the placebo has undergone a conceptual change of late.[11] The term *placebo* is rooted in Latin (*placere*) and literally means "I will please" or "placate." As late as 1960, medical dictionaries still defined placebo this way, suggesting that placebo treatment (with inert pills, for example) was a substitute for genuine therapeutic agents and procedures. What was not known, O'Connell points out, was that with rare exceptions *the "genuine" medications were themselves placebos* in a more contemporary sense of the word. This becomes apparent when we examine how the concept of the placebo has changed over the past few decades.

The first development in the history of the placebo was the discovery that pharmacologically inactive agents could duplicate the effects of their active counterparts by some sort of unknown process, and that this effect seemed powerful enough to affect all patients. The second discovery was the realization that how the placebo was administered was critical, and that pills had more power if they were provided by a sanctioned healer, such as a physician, who expressed confidence in their power. Pills don't hold much potency if they are sold over the counter by a high-school dropout at an all-night convenience store. The third discovery was that ritualistic procedures between a healer and a sufferer (without any pharmacological agents) could bring about substantial placebo effects at psychological levels.

So it turns out that big pills are better than small ones, colored ones are more effective than white ones, and big colored ones are more effective if prescribed (in Latin) than if found on the sidewalk or purchased over the counter. Injections are even more powerful, especially if given by someone in a white coat who wears a stethoscope around his or her neck—someone with several degrees on the wall and a full waiting room. They are more powerful still is if you were kept waiting a long period and if the injection was given only after a long series of expensive and complicated diagnostic tests.

What's more, research suggests that the placebo effect doesn't actually have to involve pills or injections, but that it must involve two people. The placebo effect operates whenever a sanctioned healer, who possesses the "it" which the sufferer desires, and a sufferer, who believes in the healer, get together. They must have a common faith in the healing process, and the healer must deliver a mutually acceptable prescription. Within that framework, any prescription will do.

O'Connell suggests that physicians and psychologists take a close look at the genuine placebo effect and, instead of treating it with annoyance or distain, incorporate its principles into their procedures in order to responsibly maximize change in their patients.

While the placebo effect has been demonstrated to have a significant role in all healing, it is obviously not all that there is to medicine or psychotherapy. Medicine was a "for better or for worse" proposition a century or more ago, but highly effective medications and procedures have been developed during this century. Psychotherapeutic techniques are still in an early stage of development, but they have been shown to have scientific validity and are practiced by trained and licensed professionals. But the placebo effect acts everywhere, and the fact that Dianetics, Scientology, EST, Wellsprings, and other cultlike groups do sometimes change some people's lives for the better does not suggest that they have any real scientific basis or that the consumer is in safe hands. Some consumers may come totally unglued during such treatment, and when that happens there is no one with any acceptable qualifications who can responsibly take charge. The mental health consumer should always seek out the best qualified professional, a licensed M.D. or Ph.D. from a first-rate university.

Dosage Effect and Psychotherapy: Is More Better Than Less?

When we examine research concerning the effectiveness of psychotherapy and consider the figures which reflect percentages of improvement in treatment and nontreatment groups, one thing to bear in mind is that all of this research is time-limited. Psychotherapy research projects typically last about four months, but in the offices and clinics across the country, therapy may be shorter or longer for many patients.

Psychotherapy has a dosage effect. More is better. But it is a remarkably nonlinear "more is better." Most of us show improvement very quickly, and both cost-effectiveness and improvement rates take an alarming dive after only very short treatment.

The recent *American Psychologist* special issue on psychotherapy included an analysis of the rates of patient improvement.[7] The analysis included 15 studies which concerned more than 2400 patients. Improvement rates were found to be very similar, whether based on the subjective estimates of patients after each session, or on the objective ratings of case material by clinical psychologists at the time of termination. The researchers therefore constructed a single curve which reflected the percentage of patients improved at various treatment intervals, which ranged from zero to 104 sessions (two years).

The data revealed that between 10 and 18 percent of patients can be expected to show improvement (symptom reduction) by simply making an appointment—before ever being seen by a professional. About 25 percent are improved after a single session, and more than 50 percent of all patients are improved after only eight sessions. This is very encouraging. However, after a couple of months of treatment, improvement is harder to come by. Treatment must continue for six months (25 sessions) before 75 percent of patients are improved, and for an entire year (52 sessions) to raise that figure to 85 percent. A full second year of therapy is required to bring the percentage of patients improved from 85 to 90 percent.

These are sobering figures, not only for the people who must make treatment-length policy decisions in publicly funded community clinics, but for those of us who seek help from private providers. The researchers suggest that six months of treatment (25 sessions) might be a rational time limit in publicly funded clinics which serve a very large population of patients.

The dosage effect is one of dramatically diminishing returns, but what actually happens out there in the real world of mental health providers? What sort of dose does the typical patient get? The answer depends on whether we seek help from a public clinic, or from a professional in private practice.

The recent comprehensive federal NIMH survey of mental disorders found that the average number of visits by all patients to all providers (public and private) was 4.58.[17] My students are always brought up short by hearing that the typical American sees a psychotherapist only about five times. When we take a look at those patients who are seen exclusively by professionals in private practice, a different picture emerges.

A federally funded 1980 survey revealed that one-third of all treatment was provided by psychiatrists in private practice, and that another third was provided by clinical psychologists who were also in private practice.[21] In this private arena, psychiatrists saw their patients an average of 10.9 visits, and psychologists saw theirs an average of 12.6 times. The slightly higher figure for the psychologists reflected the fact that they saw more patients in excess of 50 sessions.

The survey revealed that 64 percent of the patients seen by psychiatrists and psychologists made nine or fewer visits, and that 83 percent were seen fewer than 25 times. The most unsettling finding was that the 17 percent of the patients who were seen in excess of 24 sessions accounted for more than half of the total treatment costs paid out by the government and third-party insurers. Thus, a small minority of patients who receive long-term treatment account for the majority of the expenditure. This raises a tough social dilemma. What the figures boil down to is that, if a 24-session cap were placed on treatment paid for by the government and other insurers, the amount of third-party money (ours) available to treat the majority of troubled people (who would show rapid improvement) would be more than doubled.

But what about those of us whose improvement is very slow and necessitates long-term treatment? Some can afford it and some cannot. The survey of private-practice patient visits revealed that if we split family income at $35,000, patients whose families make less than that amount are seen an average of nine times. Those whose family income is in excess of that amount are seen an average of 18 times.

So, one important social question is: Who exactly gets the long-term treatment? Another is: Who exactly gets high-quality long-term treatment? The probability of high-quality treatment is obviously related to income. If the more affluent of us, who are functional enough to work and afford health insurance, eat up a large part of the insurance dollars, what happens to the people who really need treatment to function at all? My experience is that the nonaffluent people who suffer from serious illnesses, such as borderline personality disorders, schizophrenia, character disorders, and other disabling conditions which respond only to long-term treatment, often find themselves in the revolving doors of public clinics, frequently bounced from inexperienced intern to inexperienced intern year after year. Many live on our streets. The people who most need long-term, high-quality treatment are the ones least likely to receive it. Professional providers could bring about substantial changes in the whole insurance scenario by responsibly limiting long-term treatment to those who truly need it, and by utilizing effective short-term treatment for the majority of patients.

Apart from social issues, these data on dosage effect are important to each of us at a very personal level. In order to show improvement, some of us do, in fact, need longer treatment than others. But those of us who are still in therapy after six months, when 75 percent of all patients have shown improvement, should stop and carefully review what it was that we wanted, what we have achieved, and how the prospects look for the future before we go on.

If our goals, upon entering therapy were as slippery as "liking ourselves better," we could be in trouble, and should consider setting some very concrete, measurable behavior objectives if we go on with therapy. Stepping out of therapy for a few weeks or months to think things over is time well spent. We can always go back.

If our original goals have been met, and we have subtly moved from our goals to those of our therapist, whose notions of successful therapy may be considerably more ambitious than our own, this, too, should make us reassess before continuing. Most of us are born onto the therapeutic beach on a tidal of wave of crisis—an emotional wave which carries enough energy to smash old ways of thinking, feeling, and behaving. But such tidal courage usually recedes quickly, and sitting in the safe shade of a therapist until the next typhoon season may or may not be a good idea. We can always come back. Therapy beyond six months, for most of us, should require very serious assessment.

Dr. Nick Cummings, a well-known and respected clinical psychologist, was recently quoted in an *American Psychological Asso-*

ciation Monitor[4] article which addressed the issue of short-term therapy:

> It became clear to me that psychology is the only health field in which the patient gets what he's offered, not what he needs. If he goes to a Freudian he gets the couch. If he goes to a Jungian he's going to paint pictures. The interesting thing is this shot-gun approach works. It's just not efficient. For a phobic patient, long-term insight therapy may be about as useful as the Bubonic plague.

The article pointed out that one of the reasons short-term therapy is becoming popular is economic. Insurers are increasingly forced to limit the number of sessions they will cover, so consumers are looking for effective, less costly treatment. But more importantly there is considerable evidence that short-term or time-limited therapy is not only as effective as, but in some cases more effective than, long-term treatment. The extensive data concerning dosage and patient improvement suggest that a relatively small percentage of patients require long-term treatment, perhaps only 15 to 20 percent of them.[7] These findings suggest that the consumer should shop for psychotherapy carefully and bear in mind that brief psychotherapy is not just a small serving of the house specialty.

The brief family, cognitive, interpersonal, and analytic therapies now available follow specific procedures and require special training on the part of the therapist who wishes to add these techniques to his or her basic skills. When contrasted with long-term psychotherapies, the brief therapies are more likely to focus on the present, to clearly define the problem, to set up therapeutic goals, and to assign between-session homework tasks for the patient which will reinforce new ways of thinking, feeling, and behaving. The brief therapies may range from 10 or fewer sessions (Strategic Family Therapy) up to 20 sessions (Brief Analytic Therapy). Sessions may not be scheduled on a strict weekly basis. They may be variable or spaced out in order to allow therapeutic interventions to be tested in the patient's environment.

Data from the 15 studies included in the dosage analysis suggest that only 15 to 20 percent of patients require more than 24 sessions to improve. Dr. Gary VandenBos, a recognized and respected authority on psychotherapeutic effectiveness, states that if clinicians are well-trained, about 85 percent of patients will benefit from short-term treatment.[3]

Research and Practice

While the experts who conduct and assess research on the effectiveness of psychotherapy have contributed enormously to our knowledge about psychotherapeutic process and outcome, a recent survey reveals that practicing psychotherapists feel that such research has only limited relevance to what they do. Most continue to practice according to what their personal clinical experience dictates.[10] Such experience typically dictates that they continue to do their own chosen form of psychotherapy in the face of hundreds of studies which suggest that it is no more effective than other methods which may require less time and money. A minority of us require long-term treatment, and all of us can receive added benefits from long-term psychotherapy, but most of us neither need it nor can afford it.

There are therapists who will responsibly help us meet our own particular goals, and money well spent is money used to investigate various treatment options before making a choice. If all you had in mind was repairing the roof, think twice about acting on advice that you should add a full basement and second story to be truly happy. Perhaps you can find a qualified professional who specializes in roofs. If a roof job doesn't do it, you can always return for further work.

Finally, the consumer should be reminded that brief therapies have been demonstrated to be particularly effective in the treatment of moderate to severe depression and some of the anxiety disorders. What I am underlining here is that short-term psychotherapy is often the treatment of choice for these disorders, which most commonly afflict Americans. This is good news indeed.

The Current Status of Psychotherapy

Research on psychotherapy is complex and difficult, but psychologists and psychiatrists have made, and continue to make, substantial and responsible scientific efforts to find answers. They have demonstrated that psychotherapy is a legitimate procedure and are now investigating whether particular forms of treatment might be more or less effective for different kinds of mental disorders. With regard to the efficacy of psychotherapy we can make the following observations:

1. A substantial number of us who suffer from mental disorders experience symptom relief and improvement without treatment.
2. An analysis of hundreds of studies concerning the outcome of psychotherapy suggests that it is moderately helpful and somewhat better than no treatment.
3. All forms and kinds of psychotherapy appear at this point to be equally effective, a finding that suggests that change is largely a function of nonspecific therapist, patient, and process variables which are common to all therapeutic systems.
4. Most of us show improvement very rapidly when treated with psychotherapy. Cost-effectiveness diminishes at an ever-increasing rate after very few sessions.
5. About 85 percent of us do not require long-term psychotherapy, and since short-term therapy appears to be highly effective for the common mood and anxiety disorders which trouble most of us; we should shop for what we need rather than accept what is offered.

An overview of research concerning the incidence, causes, and treatments of mental disorders has provided a framework within which we can evaluate the effectiveness of exercise therapy. We have seen that mood and anxiety disorders are among the most common mental disorders in America, and it has been suggested that mood disorders are the most likely targets for exercise therapy.

Of particular interest is research which reveals that the commonly prescribed antidepressant drug (imipramine) and perhaps the most effective depression-specific form of psychotherapy (Beck's brief cognitive therapy) are equally effective in treating the forms of depression most commonly suffered by patients seeking outpatient treatment. The effectiveness of these treatments provides a benchmark against which we can measure exercise therapy.

The following chapter compares the effectiveness of exercise therapy to a variety of standard group and individual psychotherapies, including the depression-specific brief therapies.

Chapter 6

Exercise Therapy and Depression

I would like to suggest that running should be viewed as a wonder drug, analogous to penicillin, morphine, and the tricyclics. It has a profound potential in preventing mental and physical disease and in rehabilitation after various diseases have occurred.

—Dr. William Morgan, President
of the American Psychological
Association's Division of
Exercise and Sport Psychology

Dr. Terry Kavanagh heads up the Cardiac Department at the Toronto Rehabilitation Center, which back in 1968, with a staff of three and a handful of patients, began to use exercise as the primary treatment for postcoronary rehabilitation with the hope that the patients would lower the risk of future heart attacks by incorporating regular exercise into their lifestyles.[30] A program which gradually took the patients from walking to jogging satisfied the medical concerns of the staff, and it became the exercise treatment of choice at the center. The Toronto center now has a case load in excess of 900 and a staff of more than 50 full- and part-time professionals. The program has been very successful, with more than 75 percent of patients continuing to exercise at least three times a week eight years after discharge.

One of the many findings resulting from Kavanagh's work is that as patients become more physically fit through the jogging program, they concurrently become less depressed. Kavanagh assessed depression with the Minnesota Multiphasic Personality Inventory (MMPI), a widely accepted test of psychopathology commonly used in research. This relationship between increased fitness and decreased depression has been reported frequently.

Not so long ago a research group from Purdue University[34] compared the personalities of 11 healthy sedentary men, 40 to 60 years of age, with 11 similar men who had been running 20 to 60 minutes, three to six times a week, for the past 3 to 10 years. The scores of the men in both groups were all in the normal range, but there were differences between the personalities of the sedentary and the active men. The investigators found that the test variable that discriminated most powerfully between the two groups was the MMPI's depression scale. The physically fit middle-aged men were significantly less depressed than their sedentary brothers, who hadn't done any aerobic exercise in the past 10 years. The physically fit men were also more extraverted than were those who were sedentary. Many studies have found athletes to be on the extraverted side. Since the two groups of men did not significantly differ on the majority of the MMPI scales, and because the greatest differences were apparent on the depression scale, the investigators concluded that exercise might influence mood (feeling or affect) more than it impacts basic personality structure (the unique pattern of traits which characterizes each of us).

So what do we have here? Is it the case that extraverted and happy middle-aged men take to running joyfully through the woods and subsequently get fit? Perhaps depressed extraverts head for the woods and become both fit and happy. Or perhaps the woods are magical. Cause and effect are a matter of speculation. But this is only one of many investigations which consistently associate lower depression with increased physical fitness.

Over the years it has been demonstrated time and again that healthy college students and other adults show significant decreases in depression test scores after engaging in one or another sort of physical activity. We will discover that such research has further revealed that both the kind of activity and the amount of activity appear to be importantly associated with depression scores.

More than a decade ago Dr. Robert Brown and his colleagues at the University of Virginia began to study the relationship between exercise and moods.[9,10] They began by assessing the degree of depression among normal high school and college students both before and after 10 weeks of self-selected sports activities (which averaged 30 minutes a day, three days a week). They found that students in several groups had significantly lowered depression scores at the end of the 10 weeks of physical activity.

Most significant were the decreases shown by students in the jogging groups. Students on the wrestling team, those who engaged in mixed physical-education-class activities, and members of a high-school tennis team also showed significant depression-score reductions after 10 weeks. However, those who played softball and others who served as nonexercise controls showed no changes in depression over the same time period.

Brown and his research group then moved on to a far more ambitious project when they decided to see what effect exercise might have on students who were clinically depressed. They tested hundreds of students in psychology classes and found nearly one in five of them to be depressed. The 600 students who volunteered to participate were given a choice about whether they would remain sedentary or exercise for the next 10 weeks. Those who chose to exercise were also allowed to choose how frequently they would work out (jogging a minimum of 30 minutes either three or five times a week). Thus there were six groups of students: normals who were sedentary, who exercised three times a week, or who exercised five times a week, and three similar groups of depressed students.

Whether normal or depressed to begin with, the students who chose to remain sedentary showed no decrease in depression after the 10-week period. On the other hand, both normal and depressed students who jogged either three or five times a week showed highly significant reductions in depression scores. The reductions for the group of depressed students who jogged five times a week were quite impressive. All of the exercise groups also showed significant reductions in hostility, anxiety, and fatigue scores as well as increases in scores on scales which measured cheerfulness and energy. This study was one of the first which suggested that exercise might be related to decreased hostility, a finding that would be replicated many times in the future.

What do the results of Brown's research projects suggest? Unfortunately his findings do not prove that exercise reduces depression. Brown's very important pioneering efforts were what are called *quasi experiments*, not true experiments because the students who participated were not randomly assigned to the exercise and nonexercise (control) groups. The fact that both normal and depressed students who volunteered to be in the exercise groups reduced depression over the course of 10 weeks could be because they exercised, because they volunteered, or because of both of these factors. Perhaps volunteers are more motivated, wanting to do something about their depression more intensely. One thing which suggests that there might be some truth to the latter is that the depressed students who volunteered to exercise five times a week had initially higher depression scores than those who chose to jog only three times a week.

While Brown's results don't prove that exercise reduces depression, his findings were in the expected direction. In addition, Brown demonstrated that it was possible to get depressed individuals to jog regularly with no real supervision, and that the more depressed individuals chose to exercise more frequently. Brown, by the way, routinely assesses the moods of his students, and since the 1970s, he has tested more than 5000 men and women. This huge sample has consistently shown exercise to be related to decreased depression, anxiety, hostility, and fatigue and to improved energy and sleep. Quasi experiment or not, these are impressive numbers.

Dr. Bonnie Berger of Brooklyn College was interested in the acute (immediate) effects of exercise on depression and several other mood variables. She assessed the moods of students in two beginning swimming classes, two intermediate swimming classes, and two lecture courses at the beginning of the instructional hours.[4] Following 40 minutes of swimming or 50 minutes of lecture, the moods of all of the students were checked again. Some interesting differences emerged. The students in all four swimming classes showed very significant mood changes following their swims. They were less depressed, hostile, tense, and confused. They were also more vigorous. The changes which they showed were significantly greater that the changes evidenced by the students who had spent 50 minutes listening to a lecture.

Brown and his research team demonstrated that reduced depression seems to be associated with chronic, or repeated episodes of exercise (10 weeks of jogging), and Berger demonstrated that it is also associated with acute exercise (40 minutes of swimming) for both beginning and intermediate swimmers. The problem here is the word *associated*. Behaviors which are associated do not always involve cause and effect. Let's consider some of the problems encountered in doing controlled research on exercise and depression.

Research Design Problems and Issues

The results of the Brown and Berger studies are consistent with those of many similar investigations which have found exercise to be associated with reduced depression. The problem with these and similar studies is that we don't know whether depression scores are reduced because of exercise, because of the expectancies of the participants, because the participants chose to participate, because they chose the sport in which they would take part, or a combination of these factors.

Another problem is that research on largely normal and healthy individuals may not tell us much about those who are clinically depressed. Reductions in depression scores in normal people may simply reflect the increased feelings of well-being which regular exercisers so commonly report.

Controlled research on how exercise impacts depression is very difficult to carry out. For starters, we must find and screen large numbers of clinically depressed individuals who are willing to participate in experimental treatment, without knowing what sort of treatment they might receive. We must then randomly assign them to an exercise therapy group, to one or another sort of alternative treatment group where attention and expectancy of symptom relief are the same as for the exercise group, or to a nontreatment control group.

Then there is the matter of testing. The patient's expectancies of symptom relief should be assessed in all groups before treatment. It wouldn't do to have patients in one group harboring greater expectations that treatment will ease their depressions. Participants must also be tested for level of depression prior to the beginning of treatment, at one or more points during treatment, at the termination of treatment, and at one or more follow-up points.

Cardiorespiratory fitness should be assessed before and after treatment to verify whether or not a measurable increase in fitness actually occurred. It could be that just believing we are getting in shape might reduce our depression.

Compliance is also a problem. We must find ways to get people started in the various groups, keep them involved for the three or more months that such research normally entails, then locate them months later for follow-up assessment. It is expensive, time-consuming, and frequently frustrating. Most experiments fail to satisfy all of these criteria.

Considerable work has been done simply to find the most efficacious way to get depressed people to exercise for a half hour or more three times a week, and to keep them doing so for three months. It requires a tremendous amount of time and individual attention on the part of researchers, who must walk-run with each patient at the patient's level of fitness, keep the patient concentrated on breathing and technique, and discourage the patient from discussing personal problems and symptoms during exercise periods. If we want to assess the effects of exercise, we cannot do psychotherapy at the same time since it would contaminate the results.

Over the past 10 years, exercise therapy studies have begun increasingly to meet the sorts of experimental standards which are necessary in order to allow us to come to some tentative conclusions about whether or not exercise is a viable form of therapy for the treatment of depression. While these studies are not all above criticism, there have been many quality investigations.

Scattered among the studies I will present are some which did not include the usual no-treatment control group. These are investigations which compared the effects of exercise with one or more kinds of psychotherapy. Some investigators now argue that since the efficacy of psychotherapy has been demonstrated (it is better than no treatment), it is no longer always necessary to include a no-treatment control group. They contend that various treatment groups can be legitimately compared with one another for power and efficacy, and this argument has some merit.

Let's now consider research concerning exercise therapy and depression. It is quite diverse and interesting, answering some questions and posing others.

Baseline Studies

One increasingly popular research strategy allows individuals to serve as their own controls, by comparing their moods during both sedentary and active periods. Individuals' moods are typically assessed for several weeks prior to introducing exercise as a treatment. Frequently a nonexercise intervention, such as meditation or relaxation training, will be introduced during this "baseline" period to assess the influence of attention on normal depression levels. Exercise treatment is then introduced. Sometimes depression is assessed during the exercise phase, and it is always measured again after the exercise treatment ends. These baseline studies can be carried out with remarkable success even when only one individual is the focus of study. Let's begin with an example of a multiple (more than a single-person) baseline study.

Dr. Wesley Sime, director of the Stress Physiology Laboratory at the University of Nebraska, and a colleague studied 15 moderately depressed men and women who ranged in age from 26 to 53.[44] These individuals were assessed for depression before and after a two-week baseline period during which they met to do nonaerobic calisthenics and stretching exercises. The attention which these 15 people received during the two weeks of calisthenics and stretching had no effect on their moods. Their depression scores remained steady.

Following the two-week baseline period, these depressed men and women met four times a week to engage in a walk-run program which became gradually more demanding over the course of 10 weeks. Three individuals dropped out.

At the end of the 10 weeks the average depression scores for the remaining 12 individuals were significantly lower than they had been before the exercise program. The same was true at both 6-month and 21-month follow-ups. These results suggest that exercise *per se* reduced depression.

Two other interesting findings emerged from this experiment. One was that the men and women failed to show a significant increase in fitness (Vo_{2MAX}) after all of their fitness training. The investigators point out that this could have been due to the fact that the fitness measures were taken on a stationary bicycle. Peddling and running ask different things of our muscle groups and may differentially condition them. Perhaps a training effect would have been found if the individuals had been tested while running on a treadmill. The second interesting finding concerned the remarkable durability of the mood elevation produced by running, but follow-up interviews revealed that such durability was dependent on the patients' *continuing to exercise.* At 21 months, those who remained undepressed were either still regularly running or doing some equivalent form of aerobic exercise. Three of the individuals who were more depressed at this time had stopped exercising, and a fourth had switched to yoga. This suggests that if exercise is to permanently affect mood it may have to be a permanent addition our lifestyles.

Four women who were suffering from major depressions were recently studied in another baseline investigation.[17] These women were tested for levels of depression before and after an attention-placebo period when they did not engage in aerobic exercise. Following this period the women exercised for 30 minutes, four times a week, for six weeks. They worked out at 85 percent of their predicted maximum capacity on a stationary bicycle equipped with an ergometer which regulated exercise intensity. This constitutes a very strenuous workout. These women who suffered major depressions showed highly reliable decreases in depression (compared to baseline levels) following treatment, and the decreases were maintained at a three-month follow-up test. Increased treadmill time and lowered heart rates reflected a physical conditioning effect. While the study was not without some problems, it demonstrated that exercise is a viable prescription for adult women suffering from major depression.

Dr. Sime carried out a fascinating single-case baseline study involving a profoundly depressed suicidal patient.[44] The patient, who had failed to respond to other forms of treatment, had eventually been given electroconvulsive therapy (ECT). Following successful ECT, he had been put on a schedule of tranquilizing and antidepressant medications. He eventually became dependent on the tranquilizers and was hospitalized to undergo detox. The psychotherapist who was treating him needed assistance to deal with the patient's continuing depression. He referred the patient to Sime for adjunctive exercise therapy. The patient's moods were assessed during the eight-week period before exercise therapy and during the five exercise treatment weeks when he ran several days each week with Sime. The patient was tested daily during the five weeks of unpredictable intermittent running. He ran one, two, or three days in a row with unpredictable days off in between. Interestingly, his *depression scores showed peaks and valleys which precisely paralleled his days of activity and rest.* Sime pointed out that the effects of running on the major depression of this particular patient were acute (lasting no more than 12 to 26 hours) and that these predictably acute effects strongly suggested exercise-induced neurochemical changes in the patient's brain. Later in the chapter we will discuss just how exercise might result in such neurochemical changes.

Sime's single-case study is also of interest because he demonstrates that with proper attention by a running therapist, it is possible to treat a highly depressed and suicidal individual. He contended that the running treatment was, at least in the short run, more effective than the individual psychotherapy the man was receiving. It was the only treatment which effectively kept the depression under control.

A Pennsylvania State University graduate student carried out a baseline study which also focused on the acute or immediate antidepressant effects of running, but this time normal highly conditioned runners, rather than clinically depressed individuals, were used as experimental subjects.[48] The subjects were 20 recreational and 20 competitive runners. They were tested prior to, during, and after two days of enforced nonrunning. The runners' moods were found to be depressed during the two-day layoff, and promptly elevated again to prelayoff levels after a run on the following day. While these were not clinically depressed individuals, the results suggest that there are immediate acute mood elevations associated with running.

Exercise and Psychotherapeutic Treatment

The University of Wisconsin has been the home of considerable research on exercise therapy and depression. It was here in the 1970s that Dr. John Greist and his associates did the first pilot studies which compared exercise and psychotherapy as treatment modalities.[26,27]

In the first of the two studies, clinically depressed outpatients who came to the University Counseling Center were randomly assigned to one of three treatment groups: running therapy, individual time-limited psychotherapy (they were told it would last only 12 weeks), or individual time-unlimited dynamic insight-oriented psychotherapy (they were not initially told that it would end in 12 weeks).

Running therapy for physically unconditioned and depressed patients involves a walk-jog program where patients begin by walking, then gradually introduce increased jogging time into the exercise period until most can jog for the entire time. Jogging is simply slow running (a pace which requires more than about eight minutes per mile). Running differs from walking (and requires more effort) because after each foot plant there is a period when both of our feet are simultaneously off the ground. When we walk we always have at least one foot on the ground.

Patients in Greist's running therapy group met with running therapists three times a week for 30 or 40 minutes of exercise over a total of 10 weeks. Those in the other two groups received individual psychotherapy for 50 minutes per week for 12 weeks. Patients were tested for depression before and after treatment, as well as a year after treatment ended.

At the end of the treatment periods (10 weeks of running therapy or 12 weeks of psychotherapy), all three groups showed reductions in depression. This pioneering experiment was not a perfect one, but it suggested that running had significant potential as a treatment for moderate depression. Of significance also was that both running therapy and time-limited psychotherapy appeared to be stronger interventions in the reduction of symptomatic depression than traditional time-unlimited dynamic psychotherapy. Brief psychotherapy involves working on concrete objectives and also requires assigned tasks between sessions. Dynamic psychotherapy is an intense interpersonal therapy which is ordinarily very long-term.

Not only was running therapy as effective as traditional forms of individual psychotherapy, but it appeared to impact depression very rapidly. Six of the eight individuals in the running-therapy group were essentially free of depressed symptoms by the third week of treatment. One did not start her walk-jog program until

Week 6, and one showed no change in level of depression throughout the study.

Of the people who had received running therapy, 80 percent remained symptom-free at the time of the 12-month follow-up. By that time, half of those in the two psychotherapy groups had returned to the clinic seeking further treatment.

Because of some deficiencies in the study, Greist and his associates expanded the research five years later with improved control over a number of problematic variables. This time they invited referrals from psychiatrists in the city of Madison, Wisconsin. They treated a total of 30 depressed patients with running therapy. All but 6 of the 30 patients recovered swiftly, and of the 6 who did not, 4 never became runners.

More recently a Wisconsin research group headed up by Dr. Margorie Klein delivered an impressive experiment.[31] This time 60 very carefully screened clinically depressed individuals were randomly assigned to a running-therapy group, a meditation-relaxation therapy group, or a cognitive-interpersonal psychotherapy group.

The nonrunning therapy groups met for two hours twice a week for 12 weeks. The meditation-relaxation therapy incorporated body awareness, breathing techniques, and mastery of relaxation skills. The cognitive-interpersonal psychotherapy group was semistructured in the manner of brief therapy and was designed to help the patients recognize and modify personal maladaptive behavior patterns which had tended to perpetuate their depressions.

Individuals assigned to the running therapy group met twice a week for 45-minute walk-jog sessions which were preceded and followed by stretching and warm-up/down. Each patient met with an individual running therapist who supervised the transitional walk-to-jog program and made sure that the patient kept focused on breathing and exercise technique. Patients were not allowed to discuss their depression or personal problems during workouts. Their treatment also lasted for 12 weeks.

Not all patients completed treatment. While almost all of those assigned to the running group began treatment, only 56 percent completed the 12 weeks. This contrasts with 48 percent of those in the meditation-relaxation group and 67 percent of those in the psychotherapy group who stayed on for the full treatment period.

Losses in the two nonrunning groups were greatest as no-shows, prior to the onset of treatment. Patients in the running-therapy group were more likely to begin and then drop out later.

At the end of treatment all three groups showed significant, but not different, decreases in depression. However, differences between the groups were apparent at the time of the three-month follow-up, when members of both the running-therapy group and the meditation-relaxation therapy groups showed further gains (less depression than when treatment ended) and the psychotherapy group showed some regression back toward increased depression. Klein suggests that the increased depression following treatment on the part of the psychotherapy group might reflect the loss of group support and that the further gains on the part of members of both the running and meditation-relaxation groups might reflect self-mastery skills.

Members of the running and meditation-relaxation groups had some common experiences. Both groups focused on rhythmic body activity (breathing), self-monitoring, and the acquisition of a specific set of skills. The acquisition of specific skills, which can be independently prescribed as needed in the future, may have considerable bearing on the durability of meditation-relaxation therapy and running therapy. It may also have to do with the elevation of self-esteem which is sometimes found when people begin to exercise with regularity.

The Klein experiment revealed a few other specific trends. The runners showed a larger trend toward higher athletic self-concept (they viewed themselves more positively with regard to fitness), and the meditators showed a greater trend toward lower anxiety. The psychotherapy group showed the least improvement with regard to reduction of interpersonal complaints.

Since psychotherapy has been demonstrated to be more effective than no treatment, more and more research is being carried out which compares the effectiveness of different sorts of therapy for different sorts of mental disorders. The lack of a control group does not substantially detract from the Klein investigation. This study suggests that running therapy is as powerful as, and may be more durable than, a form of short-term group psychotherapy which has been shown to be particularly effective in the treatment of depression.

A number of graduate student theses concerning exercise and depression have come from Pennsylvania State University, where Dr. Dorothy Harris heads up the Center for Women in Sports. One such investigation involved 18 mildly depressed individuals who had been assigned to counseling. Half of these individuals, who were chosen at random, had their counseling supplemented with at least 20 minutes of exercise three times a week for 10 weeks. There were no differences in depression scores prior to treatment, but at the end of the 10 weeks, only the people in the counseling-plus-exercise group showed significant decreases in depression.[42]

Another Pennsylvania State University research team solicited volunteers through public service announcements which promised treatment for depression.[21] After the screening of a large number of applicants, 49 mild to moderately depressed men and women who were aged 19 to 62 took part. They were tested for depression at the time of screening, at a later intake interview, prior to the first day of treatment, at the end of the fifth week (midpoint) and the tenth (final) week of treatment, and again at two- and four-month follow-up.

These depressed members of the community were randomly assigned to three treatment groups. Those who received exercise therapy met in small groups of six to eight members three times a week for a 20-minute walk-run period which was preceded and followed by stretching and warm-up/down. Some were assigned to weekly individual cognitive psychotherapy. This form of psycho-therapy is a preferred and highly effective psychotherapeutic method for the treatment of moderate to major depression, and it has been demonstrated to be as effective as antidepressant medica-tion. A third group of patients received both individual psycho-therapy and exercise therapy.

Depression scores in all three groups were significantly re-duced by the third week of treatment and remained so at follow-up testing. There were no differences between the groups. Exercise alone was as effective as psychotherapy or psychotherapy plus exercise. Anxiety, anger, frustration, and confusion scores were also significantly reduced in all groups.

This experiment is interesting for at least two reasons. First, it once again demonstrates that exercise alone is as effective as psy-chotherapy for moderate depression, even when compared to the best depression treatment which psychotherapy has to offer. But what makes this experiment so very unusual is that it may be the only one where psychotherapy appeared to act as swiftly as exercise therapy, suggesting that brief cognitive therapy may indeed be the psychotherapeutic treatment of choice for depression.

One of the issues which has been debated over the years is whether or not exercise must be aerobic in order to effectively reduce depression. Some have argued that sustained strenuous aerobic exercise, which produces high internal body temperatures, the possibility of substantial neurochemical brain activity, and increased cardiorespiratory fitness, is a necessity. Others have argued that any sort of physical activity will do the job.

One study which was intended to shed light on this question involved 41 women who met the diagnostic criteria for minor or major depression.[17] These women were randomly assigned to an aerobic running group, a nonaerobic weight-lifting group, or a waiting-list no-treatment control group. Thirty-minute supervised treatment periods were scheduled four times a week for eight weeks.

At the end of the eight weeks no changes with regard to depression were observed in the waiting-list group, but both the running group and the weight-lifting groups showed significant decreases in depression scores, decreases which could be due to exercise, attention, or an increase in feelings of self-efficacy. The results would argue that exercise need not be aerobic to be associated with reduced depression. But the investigators did not report results of fitness testing, so it isn't known whether the aerobic group did in fact increase cardiorespiratory fitness. The question of whether exercise must be aerobic to decrease depression remains unanswered.

Drs. Lisa McCann and David Holmes of the University of Kansas completed an impressive study of exercise and depression which they feel meets the all of the criteria for controlled research.[37] They selected clinically depressed patients and included what they felt was a viable nonaerobic placebo group, as well as a control group. They also assessed the treatment expectancies of the patients prior to treatment and measured fitness both before and after treatment.

After testing 250 students, McCann and Holmes selected 43 mildly depressed women and randomly assigned them to three groups in an experiment which lasted 10 weeks. The women were told that the tests which they had taken had revealed that they might be experiencing some problems with stress in their lives (rather than that they were moderately depressed) and that the experiment was one which investigated stress management techniques.

One group of women engaged in strenuous exercise (a class in aerobic dance, jogging, and running) for one hour twice a week. The placebo group was told that relaxation exercises preceded by mild exercise (a five-minute walk) were helpful in managing stress. After instruction in relaxation exercises they were told to combine a brief walk with 20 minutes of relaxation exercise four days a week. The third group of women was told that there was currently no room to schedule them and that they would have to wait to participate in the treatment.

The three groups showed no differences with regard to their expectations of treatment success and no differences in average depression levels at the time of screening. However, all three groups showed significantly decreased depression scores by the time they showed up for the pretreatment meeting. Expectation of depression relief appears to be a powerful force. You may recall a study in the previous chapter which discovered that simply making an appointment to see a psychotherapist could result in symptom relief for nearly one in five patients.

When treatment began, the three groups sorted themselves out. By Week 5 the aerobic group had showed significantly greater reductions in depression scores than the placebo group. The differences were even greater by Week 10. The aerobic group also showed significantly increased physical fitness as measured by Cooper's 12-minute walk-run test of aerobic capacity (the greatest distance one can cover in 12 minutes is converted to a reasonably good estimate of cardiorespiratory fitness).

McCann and Holmes see these results as strong evidence that aerobic exercise per se is a viable treatment for mild depression. A question could be raised as to whether the students in the non-aerobic placebo group received attention equivalent to those in the aerobic group. A 10-week course within a class of rhythmic aerobics where there is an instructor and fellow participants is not the same thing as personally administering one's own daily relaxation exercises on the basis of verbal and written instructions delivered at the onset of the 10-week treatment period.

Of the many studies discussed this far, only three have included patients who suffered from major depression, and in some cases the criteria for classification were not as rigorous and as clearly delineated as those spelled out in the American Psychiatric Association's *Diagnostic and Statistical Manual* (DSM-III). Lets take a look at an important experiment which was conducted with men and women who not only met the DSM-III criteria for major depression, but were so depressed that all were hospitalized and many were medicated with antidepressants. This research was conducted by Dr. Egil Martinsen, director of the Modum Bads Nervesanatorium in Norway.[36]

Martinsen's 49 patients ranged in age from 17 to 60. The duration of the current major depressive episode was in excess of 6 months for 33 of these men and women. The 49 patients had had an average of eight previous depressive episodes, with their initial episode typically occurring about eight years prior to their current hospitalization. These were severely depressed individuals. Martinsen wondered whether they would exercise, and whether exercise would impact such incapacitating depression.

He randomly assigned these 49 individuals to exercise and control groups. All 49 received standard treatment, which included both individual psychotherapy and occupational therapy, but half of them underwent a nine-week exercise program which included walking, jogging, bicycling, skiing, and swimming at 50 to 70 percent of maximal aerobic capacity for one hour, three times a week. All patients were tested for depression and fitness (bicycle ergometer) before the nine-week exercise program began, and at three, six, and nine weeks.

At the end of the nine-week treatment period, the patients who added exercise to their regular treatments were found to have significantly higher fitness scores and significantly lower depression scores than the patients who did not exercise.

The study did have some minor problems. For example, the random assignment of patients resulted in unequal numbers of individuals who were taking antidepressant medication in the two groups. Antidepressant medication was used throughout the research period by 38 percent of the exercisers and 73 percent of the nonexercisers. What effect this had is not known. Members of the exercise group also received a greater amount of attention and may have had greater expectancies of symptom relief with this extra treatment program. Two things, however, make this study worthy of our attention. The first concerns fitness. There was a very strong correlation between increased fitness and lower depression scores for the men in this study, but not for the women, where the correlation was low enough to be insignificant. Martinsen argues that these findings suggest that the antidepressant effects of exercise may have multiple causes. We will shortly discuss some of theories concerning the various ways in which exercise might impact depression.

The second significant feature of this investigation is that it demonstrates that it is possible to use exercise as a form of antidepressant therapy in an institutional setting with men and women who currently suffer from major depression and have a history of multiple major depressive episodes. Such severely depressed individuals will in fact exercise and can exercise safely under supervision, even when taking antidepressant medication.

Conclusions and Theoretical Hypotheses

These many investigations consistently support the notion that exercise therapy can serve as an effective primary or adjunctive treatment for clinically depressed outpatients who suffer from moderate and major depressions, as well as for institutionalized patients suffering very severe recurrent major depression. The magnitude of change which results from exercise therapy by itself is as great as that associated with a variety of standard group and individual psychotherapies, some of which, in turn, have been shown to be as effective as antidepressant drug therapy. In addition, several experiments demonstrate that exercise therapy reduces depressive symptoms very rapidly, usually within three to five weeks.

What is so very amazing about research on moderate to major depression is that symptom reduction is associated with such a vast array of treatments. Aerobic and possibly nonaerobic exercise, a wide variety of individual and group psychotherapies, meditation-relaxation training, antidepressant drugs, and even no treatment have all been associated with significant reductions in such depressions. While treatments of one sort or another are consistently superior to no-treatment, there is as yet no convincing evidence that any one of them produces a greater magnitude of change than any other over the course of three or four months of treatment. How can such diverse treatments yield such similar results?

For starters, all forms of treatment share some features. Motivated patients, who expect to be helped, are paid attention to by kind and helpful experts who deliver a prescription in which both the patient and the healer have faith. The prescription may be pills, exercise, meditation, or psychotherapy. These common features, which together constitute a placebo effect, may account for a considerable part of the depression reduction which is associated with such a wide of diversity of interventions.

It may also be that each of these various treatments has an independent contribution which uniquely functions to further impact depression. For example, both antidepressant drugs and exercise are associated with more rapid symptom reduction than that associated with most psychotherapies. Exercise and meditation-relaxation training have also been associated with depression reduction which appears to be durable, in some cases more durable than that associated with psychotherapy.

Bearing in mind that the relevant research is scattered and preliminary in nature, let's consider some of the hypotheses which deal with just how exercise might uniquely function in the reduction of depression.[45]

Physiological Explanations

When thinking about the antidepressant effects of exercise, the most obvious point of departure is to look for a *physiological* explanation. Exercise, for example, results in an increase in blood flow and oxygenation to our central nervous system, and exercise therapy is unique in that a sufficient frequency, intensity, and duration produces a wide range of significant physiological changes, including enhanced cardiorespiratory fitness.

A physiological theory goes something like this. If building a big, efficient heart results in a decreased physiological response to physical stress, it may also result in a decreased response to psychological stress, which in turn may reduce depressive reactions to such stress. That seems like an impressive number of bridges to cross, and there are some problems with this line of thinking.

One problem is that there is no consistently demonstrated relationship between increased cardiovascular fitness and reduced depression. We just read of how Martinsen found that men suffering from major depression exhibited such a relationship, but that women did not. In addition, several of the studies which have been discussed in this chapter demonstrate that exercise significantly reduces depression in about half the time (3 to 5 weeks) necessary to reliably produce an aerobic fitness effect (8 to 10 weeks). Finally, it remains to be demonstrated that cardiovascular fitness can reliably decrease physiological responses to psychological stress. At this point, broad physiological explanations for how exercise functions to reduce depression don't hold together.

Biochemical Explanations

Perhaps the most intriguing hypotheses concerning exercise and depression center on *biochemical* activity. Most of us have heard of the "runner's high" and the euphoria-producing brain chemical called beta endorphin. We have all been warned that we could get hooked on the endogenous (internally produced) opiates which become active when we exercise. We could become sneaker junkies who ruin our health and family life, compulsively driven to the running trails for our daily hit of beta endorphin. But there is a difference between myth and reality.

It's sad but true that many runners have never experienced a euphoric high, and those who report having done so don't consistently experience it. If you ask large groups of runners whether they have ever experienced such a high while running, the percentage who say yes ranges from as low as 10 percent[43] to as high as 78 percent.[32] And, of course, there is no evidence that those who report experiencing such euphoria are experiencing anything like that produced by a hit of heroin. However, the chemical structure of the beta endorphin which we produce endogenously is very similar to that of opium and is 20 to 50 times more potent, and there are some very seductive research findings which suggest that beta endorphin may well be involved in the exercise-mood formula.

An analysis of brain tissue in rats, for example, reveals significant increases in opiate-receptor-site occupancy after they have been forced to run in an activity wheel or swim in cold water.[39,50] It has also been demonstrated that mice that work out regularly can become swimming junkies. They show the same sort of dependency as that produced by morphine, exhibiting typical withdrawal symptoms when injected with the antagonist drug naloxone, a drug which interferes with beta endorphin locking into opiate receptor sites.[12]

While science has advanced to where routine measurements of what happens in the brains of rats following exercise can be conducted, for obvious reasons we cannot directly examine human brain tissue to assess beta-endorphin-receptor-site occupancy. Even trying to assess indirectly what happens with regard to neurotransmitter activity in our brains is difficult.

Beta endorphin is active within our brains as well as out in various other peripheral systems in our bodies. Our blood-brain barrier is a biochemical filter which regulates which substances pass between our bloodstream and our brain's neurons, so the contents of blood samples do not directly reflect what is happening in our brains. We simply don't know whether endorphin levels outside our brains covary (rise and fall in a parallel manner) with those within the brain, where important pleasure and pain centers reside. Research on the effects of exercise on beta endorphin levels in human beings has been restricted to measuring levels of beta endorphin and its metabolites (enzymes break down or degrade neurotransmitters into metabolites) in our peripheral blood, the blood out beyond the blood-brain barrier. Bearing in mind that such measures do not accurately reflect what is happening in our brains, let's have a look at what happens to beta endorphin levels in our peripheral blood when we exercise.

Dr. Daniel Carr[11] and a large group of colleagues from a number of Boston medical facilities recruited seven unconditioned women for a rigorous and increasingly intense physical training program which lasted two months. Since simply having blood drawn can elevate beta endorphin levels, blood-plasma endorphin levels were assessed during a preexercise baseline period. The women then began to exercise for an hour a day on six days of each week. Their plasma endorphin levels following exercise rose dramatically, elevating from 57 percent above normal during the first week, and on up to 145 percent above normal by the end of the eight-week period. This research suggests that there is an *acute* or immediate response to exercise (beta endorphin levels elevate after only a couple of minutes of exercise according to Dr. Walter Bortz II[6]) and also a *chronic* effect, which builds over time. The above-average endorphin levels produced by exercise in these women progressively rose as the weeks of increasingly vigorous exercise continued.

Plasma endorphin levels have also been shown to elevate in response to running.[5,18,19] Bortz[6] has found this to be true in ultra-marathoners competing in the arduous Western States 100 mountain race, as has Otto Appenzeller[1,2] who has assessed levels of endorphin in trekkers in the high Himalayas and runners in long-distance mountain races here in the American Southwest. Appenzeller reassures us that the chronic response of endorphin to continued exercise is self-limiting. That is, endorphin levels don't continue forever to spiral upward in individuals who endurance-train over months or years. While Carr found levels to increase up to 145 percent above normal in his previously unconditioned women research subjects, Appenzeller tells us that levels of plasma endorphin seem to peak at around 100 percent above normal in experienced marathoners and stay at that level during long-distance races. If this were not the case, we might have exercise junkies, with smiles of ecstasy on their faces, sitting and staring vacantly along our roadsides.

There is another interesting avenue of research which has been pursued by other investigators. It involves the use of the opiate antagonist naloxone. Naloxone is a drug which interferes with beta endorphin binding at its receptor sites, reducing the euphoric and pain-reducing effects of beta endorphin (and other opiates). A small injection of naloxone, for example, can save the life of someone who has overdosed on heroin by binding to the receptor sites normally occupied by opiates and bringing the patient out of a coma state. A drug like naloxone, which interferes with the effects of beta endorphin, has application for research designed to determine whether exercise increases levels of beta endorphin in our brains.

One group of researchers measured pain sensitivity in experienced runners, then gave them an injection of either naloxone or an inert placebo prior to a one-mile run. Pain sensitivity was then reassessed. Presumably those who received the naloxone (which blocked opiate receptor sites) would be more sensitive to pain than those whose receptor sites were open to receive pain-relieving endorphins. The investigators originally found no support for the endorphin hypothesis, but when they replicated their experiments with larger naloxone doses, the hypothesis was supported: individuals who had received substantial doses of naloxone were more sensitive to pain and scored higher on depression scales after exercise than those who had received placebo injections.[28]

A second research group did a similar experiment, but instead of measuring pain sensitivity, they measured anxiety levels in experienced runners prior to and after an hour's baseline run. The runners then completed the same run after having received either naloxone or placebo injections. Anxiety was reduced under both naloxone and placebo conditions in the same manner as it had been reduced during the baseline run. The investigators concluded that either beta endorphin does not mediate mood change or the naloxone dosage had been inadequate.[35]

At present, the hypothesis that exercise-produced endorphins result in mood alteration remains tenable. Morgan has pointed out that even if endorphin levels in our brains and in our peripheral systems do not covary, changes in peripheral opiate levels (which reflect adrenal gland activity) can theoretically affect our emotional states.[38]

While changes in endorphin levels appear to be related to feelings of well-being and euphoria, it has not been satisfactorily demonstrated that they play a central role in depression. There are some other neurotransmitters which clearly do, and regulatory problems within these other systems provide us with two models for biochemical depression.

The Aminergic Hypothesis

Many theorists and researchers see the catecholamine (dopamine and norepinephrine) and indolamine (serotonin) neurotransmitter systems as central in depression.[22,26,38,41,52]

The aminergic hypothesis suggests that there are two forms of biogenic depression which are associated with insufficiencies within the norepinephrine and serotonin systems, and there is now a sizable amount of human and animal research which lends credence to this line of thinking.

Studies have shown that antidepressant drugs such as imipramine which activate the serotonergic and norepinephrine systems in our brains can effectively reduce depressive symptoms in many of us.[23,24] It was pointed out in Chapter 3 that some depressed individuals can effectively reduce symptoms by simply ingesting larger than normal amounts of ordinary dietary amines, such as tyrosine and L-tryptophan. These amines, which are found in a variety of the foods we regularly consume, are precursors to norepinephrine and serotonin. Tyrosine is transported through our blood-brain barrier and is used to manufacture norepinephrine. L-Tryptophan can similarly impact serotonin levels in our brains.

Electroconvulsive therapy also increases aminergic (dopamine, norepinephrine, serotonin) neurotransmitter activity in our brains.[25] Other investigators have found decreased excretion of serotonin and norepinephrine metabolites in some depressed individuals.[20] While the evidence is necessarily indirect, there is substantial research which suggests that serotonin- and norepinephrine-system insufficiencies are *associated* with two kinds of biogenic depression.[22]

It is important to keep in mind that the neurochemistry of depression is profoundly complex and is only beginning to be understood. It was pointed out in Chapter 4, for example, that the effectiveness of antidepressant drugs is directly related to their capacity to block cholinergic receptors and to reduce the sensitivity of the norepinephrine-coupled adenylate cyclase system in the limbic forebrain and frontal cortex. It was also suggested that the antidepressant effects of drugs which elevate serotonin activity are most probably the result of the actions of the first metabolites of these drugs which serve to elevate norepinephrine activity and impact postsynaptic systems. Functional dopamine activity was also found to be reduced in some depressed patients.

Let's now examine research which considers the possibility that exercise can somehow mimic the effects of antidepressant drugs by activating the serotonin and norepinephrine systems within our brains. Once again, all such research must be indirect, since we do not have direct assess to human brains.

It is possible to arrange the environments of rats so that some are forced to become long-distance runners or swimmers. Once we have physically conditioned rodent athletes, we can compare their brain tissues with those of sedentary rats. Rat athletes have significantly higher levels of both serotonin and norepinephrine in their brains following workouts.[3,7,8]

Other studies have shown that rats that suffer from stress-induced depression have lower norepinephrine levels in their brains[52] and that regular swimming and running can reduce emotionality in rats.[47,51]

Research teams have found that regular exercise alters plasma and urinary levels of norepinephrine and its metabolites in humans.[16,40] Blood plasma and urinary levels of norepinephrine have been shown to increase to two to six times the normal levels during acute exercise[29] and it has been reported that plasma norepinephrine and dopamine levels in experienced runners competing in a marathon elevate three times above normal and maintain that level until the 26-mile race ends, when they bounce to about six times above normal before dropping back down to normal in an hour or so.[1]

As in the case of endorphins, we just don't know what happens with regard to norepinephrine and serotonin levels in human brains as a result of exercise. But in spite of the fact that evidence is indirect, the hypothesis that exercise ameliorates depression by activating the norepinephrine and serotonergic systems is a compelling one.

Human neuroendocrine studies, investigations of urinary and cerebospinal fluid amine metabolites, and studies on the effects of antidepressant drugs all suggest that disregulation of the serotonergic and norepinephrine systems is associated with depression in some individuals.[22] Investigations of the effect of exercise on human depression which have been considered in this chapter would seem to suggest that the effects of exercise are short-lived for many of us, and that exercise must be maintained if its antidepressant effects are to be perpetuated.[44,48] Sime's work with the depressed suicidal patient, which we discussed earlier in this chapter, caused him to report that, although his patient received regular cognitive psychotherapy, exercise was the most potent acute antidepressant agent. The dramatic parallel between exercise and depression levels (exercise's antidepressant effect appeared to last no more than 12 to 26 hours) caused Sime to suggest that a biochemical aminergic explanation could best account for these findings. Sime's second study of 15 depressed patients also suggested that for exercise to be an effective antidepressant after treatment ends, it must be maintained. The fact that exercise so closely mimics the effects of the antidepressant medications, usually relieving symptoms in three to five weeks, also lends support to the aminergic hypothesis.

The aminergic hypothesis is necessarily based on indirect evidence, and the biochemical processes involved in exercise and depression are certainly far more complicated than what is assumed in this oversimplified hypothesis. But the aminergic theory of exercise-induced mood elevation stands as a highly plausible one.

When I discuss this notion with sedentary friends, they say, "What a shame that a month or two of exercise therapy doesn't permanently eliminate depression." My standard response is, "What a shame that Americans have become unnaturally sedentary and unnaturally depressed."

Cognitive Hypotheses

When we first begin to exercise strenuously, it is often so painful that it is difficult even to think about all of the things which depress and trouble us. Thoughts of catching our breath or stopping to ease our pain fully occupy us. But when we become well conditioned and can take off for a 10-mile run without forethought, it takes no great talent to both run and obsess about our miseries. However, it has recently been discovered that we may be less likely to think about unpleasant things while we run. Such research forms the basis of a cognitive hypothesis of how exercise might reduce depression.

A number of studies has now demonstrated that how we feel (our mood) differentially affects the accessibility of positive and negative thoughts.[13,33,46] It's been shown, for example, that learned material is more easily recalled if we are in the same emotional state as when we learned it.[14] What this suggests is that when we are depressed we are more likely to retrieve depressing memories and associations, setting up a self-feeding, circular mechanism. Depressing rumination feeds on itself and may carry us ever further into the depths.

These sorts of findings lend credence to the contention of endurance athletes who claim that is impossible to exercise hard and long and be depressed. Strenuous exercise and depression are poles apart in terms of feeling states. Exercise is a highly energized state of arousal—a mood state which may make it more difficult to retrieve negative memories and associations. Thus, exercise may be a viable wedge to break into a ruminative negative thought system—one which will increase the accessibility of positive thoughts. Even apart from strenuous exercise, it has long been folk wisdom that depressed people will feel better "if we can just get them up and moving."

The cognitive hypothesis is an exciting and tenable one, but it has recently run into trouble.[15] It appears clear that an emotional-context effect does exist and does affect memory, but the relationship between emotion and memory may be less obvious than was originally thought. Attempts to experimentally replicate early findings have failed, and mixed findings have raised more questions than they have answered. It appears, for example, that emotional arousal biases judgment and perception. Individuals who have just finished strenuous exercise (soccer or tennis) rate quotations and pictures of people as being more joyful than do individuals who have not exercised. The relationship between mood and memory needs considerable experimental attention before we can say how it might help to explain the consistent association which exists between exercise and depression reduction.

Apart from our moods' differentially affecting what sorts of memories we retrieve, there is another possible avenue of change to be considered within the framework of the antagonistic physiological states which characterize depression and exercise. We sometimes embrace strenuous exercise as the final desperate attempt to relieve a crippling depression which has failed to respond to other interventions. When we are forced, by physical pain and exhaustion, to stop after a first desperate and acute bout of vigorous exercise, our train of thoughts might go something like this: "My God, I haven't thought about my problems for 20 minutes!" Gasp. "If I did it today I can do it tomorrow, maybe for even 25 minutes." The emphasis here should be on the *I*. Strenuous exercise is not something you can purchase and not something an expert does to you, for you, or with you. It is your very own virtually cost-free, self-administered, guaranteed intervention. Each day you can lace on your two sneakers, the one named "Control" and the other named "Hope." Helplessness and hopelessness breed depression. An internal locus of control breeds hope which can lead us out of depression. This line of thinking leads us to notions of self-efficacy.

Self-Efficacy and Skills Mastery

Drs. Zeiss and Munoz wrote an interesting article which addressed the question of why so many forms of treatment successfully reduce depression with equal effectiveness.[53] In discussing nonspecific treatment variables they suggested that the criteria necessary for success were (1) a rational providing structure which helps patients believe that they can control their own behavior; (2) the teaching of significant skills to the patient; (3) an emphasis on independent use of these skills and personal goal attainment; and (4) attribution of improved mood to the patient's personal skills mastery. This sounds very familiar and may help explain why, of the many brands of psychotherapy, brief cognitive therapy might be particularly effective with depression. Brief cognitive psychotherapy, meditation-relaxation therapy, and exercise therapy all incorporate these elements.

Support for the hypothesis that skills mastery and self-efficacy are significant nonspecific variables in depression reduction is found in research discussed in this chapter. A three-month follow-up revealed that four women who had reduced major depressions by exercising on stationary bicycles for several weeks maintained those gains.[17] Another investigation revealed that three months after treatment ended, patients who had received running therapy or meditation-relaxation therapy had actually continued to reduce their depressions, while those who had been in group therapy had shown a tendency to become more depressed again.[31] Both running and meditation-relaxation therapy incorporate the learning of self-monitoring, body-awareness skills which involve concentration on muscle groups and breathing techniques. Knowing that we have an "antidepressant skill in the bank" to be put into use next time we are visited by depression could add to our permanent feeling of self-sufficiency.

Some Thoughts on the Theories

It's important to bear in mind that these theories, which attempt to account for exactly how exercise functions to reduce the symptoms of depression are simply theories at this juncture. The validity of each rests on experimental work which has yet to be done. It may well turn out to be the case that all of these hypotheses will be shown to play a legitimate role in explaining the antidepressant effects of exercise.

Some of the research which I have presented seems to support one theory and reject others. This is not surprising when we consider the complexity of the questions which researchers are attempting to answer. The causes for depression are many, and the personalities of depressed individuals are diverse.

For example, the question of whether exercise has to be continuous following the termination of an exercise-therapy treatment period has not yet been resolved. Some of us seem to remain permanently free of depressive symptoms after a few weeks or months of exercise therapy even though we stop exercising, while others of us must continue to exercise if we wish to avoid becoming depressed again. This is not surprising when we recognize that each of us is biogenically unique, that each of us has also learned our own unique ways of coping adaptively or maladaptively to the world around us, and that of each us dwells within a unique environment which plays a role in determining the amount and kind of stresses with which we must contend.

Some of us become depressed as a result of a significant life event, such as the loss of an important relationship or a job. Such normal depressions are almost always self-limiting and eventually terminate whether or not they are treated with psychotherapy, drugs, or exercise. Thus, some of us might take antidepressants, see a psychotherapist, or engage in exercise therapy and appear to permanently end a depression which would have ended anyway. "Permanent" cures may frequently fall into this category.

Others of us can suffer aminergic system disregulation and insufficiency as a result of chronic physical or psychological stress. An unremitting physical illness or disability or unresolved domestic, job, or relationship problems can overwork, exhaust, and deplete aminergic systems which are constantly activated during such long-term stress. Beginning an exercise program could be only one of many significant decisions and lifestyle changes we bring to bear in order to confront the causes of the stress. Such changes could remove the causes of the stress and the resulting aminergic insufficiency, ending the depression as well as the need to continue exercising. This is another circumstance where some of us could appear to be "permanently cured" by a period of exercise therapy.

It is also the case that we are not all created equal. Some of us may have been born with, and must live with, aminergic systems which are somehow insufficient, and an aminergic theory best accounts for why exercise reduces our biogenic brand of depression. If our aminergic insufficiency is substantial, we may have to make exercise a permanent addition to our lives, unless we want to live with all of the problems associated with constantly medicating ourselves with antidepressants.

Others of us whose biogenic predisposition to depression involves less severe aminergic insufficiency might have to exercise only during those periods when stress further disregulates our amine systems, causing us to become depressed.

If future research is going to determine just exactly how exercise functions to reduce depression it will be necessary to carefully select patients, taking into account not only the severity of their depressions, but also the etiology or causes of those depressions. If all people who are depressed are lumped together in this sort of research, we may be unable to answer the questions we have concerning exercise and depression. It seems highly likely that exercise therapy will impact different individuals in different ways. Some of us may need to self-medicate disregulated aminergic systems either periodically or continually, while others of us may be more strongly impacted by the cognitive or self-mastery elements which exercise therapy offers.

Summing Up

A review of research concerning the viability of exercise therapy as a treatment for depression certainly allows optimism. While more work will be required to address many unanswered questions, what has been done is very promising and encouraging. Just exactly how exercise functions to reduce depression remains the focus of several tenable hypotheses, all of which may have some validity. However, it is increasingly apparent that exercise therapy is associated with depression reduction, and that it appears to have a number of strengths and weaknesses.

Magnitude. Exercise therapy reduces the symptoms of moderate and major depression as effectively as a wide variety of individual and group psychotherapies, some of which, in turn, have been shown to reduce depressive symptoms as effectively as a tricyclic antidepressant.

Effect Speed. Exercise may be the only treatment available which offers immediate mood-elevating effects. In addition, clinically depressed individuals who exercise are usually symptom-free within three to five weeks. In this latter regard, exercise mimics the effects of antidepressant drug therapy. Brief cognitive psychotherapy, which has been developed specifically to impact depression, may act as rapidly, but other standard conventional psychotherapies appear to act more slowly than exercise and antidepressant drug therapies.

Stability. One of the strengths of exercise therapy is that its effects appear to be durable. There is some evidence that exercise must be continued with regularity following treatment in order to effectively control depression, but this may depend on the biochemistry of the patient and the cause of the depression.

Universality. The effectiveness of exercise therapy has thus far been demonstrated with adult outpatients and inpatients diagnosed with moderate to very severe major depression. It has been safely used with patients who were taking antidepressant medication. Its effectiveness has not yet been tested with children or bipolar patients.

Side Effects. In contrast to antidepressant drugs, which have many negative side effects, exercise therapy results in a very large number of positive psychological and physiological benefits. This broad spectrum of benefits constitutes one of exercise therapy's great strengths.

Prevention. While there is an absence of direct experimental evidence that regular endurance training diminishes the probability of depressive episodes and reduces the intensity of such episodes, data suggest that this might prove to be an additional strong point.

Safety. Some form of exercise can be safely engaged in by almost everyone, including those of us with morbid (life-endangering) obesity or who are in a wheelchair or recovering from a cardiac infarction. Supervision of exercise programs is obviously required for those of us who suffer these or other sorts of risks. There is currently no evidence that regular exercise inherently leads to pathological exercise-dependence. This issue will be considered in a later chapter.

Acceptability. While exercise is available to nearly everyone, not everyone is willing to accept or comply with the prescription. About 50 percent drop out of exercise programs within six months, and the dropouts are usually those who could most benefit from exercise: overweight people and those who smoke. However, exercise-therapy dropout rates are highly variable, and all forms of therapy have serious problems with dropouts.

Variety. Exercise can be solitary, social, competitive, or easygoing. There are a wide variety of sports which are season-appropriate for all of us, wherever we live. Treatment variety is a significant strength of exercise therapy.

Cost-Effectiveness. Exercise is cheap. Walking and running are basically free—we all need shoes. One visit to a psychotherapist costs more than a year's supply of high-quality running shoes.
Convenience. Exercise is as near as your front door.

It is time now to move on to a consideration of just how exercise can be put to work to ease our depressions. I will do this in two related chapters.

The chapter which follows is written in part with physicians and mental health professionals in mind, people who may wish to prescribe exercise as an adjunctive treatment for their depressed patients. However, the chapter includes considerable information which nonprofessional readers can directly apply to their own lives or family members who are depressed and could benefit from exercise.

A chapter which will specifically address how we can self-prescribe exercise to impact our own moods will follow later in the book.

Chapter 7

The Exercise Prescription for Depression

> Better to hunt in fields for health unbought,
> Than fee the doctor for nauseous draught.
> The wise, for cure, on exercise depend; . . .
>
> —John Dryden

This chapter begins with a case which illustrates the combined application of two very potent therapeutic interventions which appear to have a significant interactive effect.

The first intervention, exercise therapy, is prescribed to deal with the patient's depression, anxiety, and insomnia. The second intervention, symptom prescription, is brought to bear on the patient's obsessive guilt rumination, a symptom which is remarkably resistant to most psychotherapeutic interventions. I include sections of dialogue which transpired during a few therapy sessions so that the reader can become acquainted with the theory and application of symptom prescription within the actual context of treatment.

I will preface this presentation with a cautionary note. On the surface, the notion of prescribing symptoms (instructing a patient to purposefully schedule or do more of the very symptomatic behavior he or she is trying to get rid of) seems quite radical or even nonsensical. However, symptom prescription is a powerful intervention which forms the very core of some highly effective brief psychotherapeutic systems, and it is not thoughtlessly employed.[4]

Professional psychotherapists do not, for example, suggest that hopeless and depressed patients feel even more hopeless and depressed, that an individual who is concerned about excessive drinking should drink even more, or that someone who has periodically thought about suicide should seriously consider it.

Symptom prescription is a special kind of "resistance utilization" technique, which is designed to utilize the power of the patient's resistance (to change or be told what to do) to reduce his or her symptomatic behaviors. The case should give the reader a feel for how this technique is employed, why it has such power, and why the combination of exercise therapy with symptom prescription has special significance in this particular circumstance.

Marty: A Case Study

Marty did not look at all well as he dumped himself into my office chair for our first visit. He seemed washed out and without energy. The clouded and emotionally flat eyes which silently regarded me didn't look as though they had harbored hope for a very long time. I remember sitting there in the early silence, feeling the weight of his despair, but drawn toward him. I found myself leaning forward in my chair, legs apart, elbows on my knees, chin resting in my clasped hands as I looked into his face. After a few moments I unclasped my hands and extended my open palms toward him before pulling them back to my chest in a silent invitation for him to give his troubles to me. He sized me up a little longer, then opened with, "If it weren't for my two sons I don't know if I would want to go on living."

Marty said that I was probably his last hope. He had run out of resources. He'd talked with friends, been prescribed medication by his physician, and seen a psychotherapist for a few sessions, but nothing had given him relief from the pervasive guilt and uncontrolled rumination which seemed to crowd everything else out of his consciousness. In his mind he was certain that he had been responsible for his wife's suicide, the subsequent distress of his two boys, and the unending downward spiral of his entire life.

As Marty spelled out what had happened during the past six months, it was apparent that some sort of powerful intervention had to be made at once for he was becoming increasingly dysfunctional. His two boys, who were in first grade and kindergarten, had developed serious difficulties in school, had lost their friends, and were suffering from nightmares. Marty was unable to parent them adequately. He was also in danger of losing his job. His entire accumulated sick leave had been used, and he had taken two leaves of absence. He was unable to concentrate on his work, and even commuting between work and home had become almost too much for him. His obsessions were so powerful and pervasive that he would "lose himself" in thought and "come to" feeling disoriented. Marty's support system had slowly eroded during the months since his wife's death. One by one his friends had fallen away, unable to bear up under the weight of his guilt and his constant obsessions. His friends' gradually fading from sight without explanation added to the negative feelings Marty had about himself. They, too, must secretly believe that he was to blame.

His marriage had been a troubled one, but each time he had brought up the topic of a separation or divorce, his wife told him that she would kill herself if he ever left her. On two occasions when he had planned to go backpacking with friends, she had had to be taken to an emergency room the night before he was scheduled to leave. She had refused help. Finally, when Marty became desperate, he had told her that he was going away for a weekend to try to sort things out. Shortly before he returned that Sunday evening, his two boys found their mother dead in the bathtub.

Marty's long story ended when he said, "Ever since she died, everyone has been telling me that I shouldn't feel guilty. When my therapist told me the same thing, I gave up and quit. I figured no one understood."

I told him that I wanted to spend some extra time with him that day and asked him to excuse me while I left for a few minutes to see if I could reschedule my next appointment.

When I returned I sat for a minute or two, then told him that I was sure that all of his friends, his physician, and his therapists had earnestly tried to help, but that maybe there was nothing any of them could really have done during that six-month period. Perhaps they didn't understand how truly guilty he felt. I added that I would probably have felt the same way he was feeling. He quickly raised his eyes to mine with a "say more" look on his face. It was the most energetic and encouraging thing I had seen the entire hour.

I went on, "If there is anything I have learned in my life it is that we always feel exactly what we are supposed to feel. I have a deep faith that what we feel always makes sense."

I watched Marty's eyes fill momentarily. His shoulders dropped and he emptied his lungs with a hushed long rush of air. It was awhile before he began breathing and looked up again.

I went on. "It sounds to me like all of your friends and your therapist gave you well-meaning advice, and that you've done your best with it. I am wondering if, now after six months of such a diligent effort to stop feeling responsible and guilty, you would be willing to give it up as a lost cause and try something else."

"I'm willing to try almost anything," said Marty.

After more than 30 years of doing psychotherapy there are a few basic principles in which I have deep faith. These principles involve our universal predisposition to resist change, and their fundamental power seems to cut beneath anything else within my professional grasp. The foundation is Dr. Milton Erickson's principle of *resistance utilization*, the notion that one always accepts what the patient offers and uses that offering on the patient's behalf.[2] Marty had brought me an obsession with guilt, something which everyone else had rejected. For starters, I knew that I must accept Marty's guilt and use it to his benefit.

Jay Haley, strategic therapist and cofounder of the Family Therapy Institute in Washington, D.C.,[5,6,7] Dr. Paul Watzlawick and the strategic therapy group at the Mental Research Institute in Palo Alto,[3,12] Dr. Mara Palazzoli of the Center for the Study of Families in Milan, Italy,[10] and others[1] have embraced Erickson's resistance utilization principle and his notions concerning reframing. Haley tells us that if you wish to change a person's inconsequential behavior, you ask that person directly to do something else, but that if the behavior you wish to change is of any significance whatsoever, you ask the person to keep on doing it and make the task an unpleasant one. He calls it the "benevolent ordeal."

If we are going to gain control over patients' symptoms by telling them that they should actually engage in more of the very thing they are trying to get rid of, we must be masters at reframing that unwanted behavior. Without skillful reframing there is no hope that we can sell the prescription and make the benevolent ordeal work. My job was to convince Marty that he wasn't feeling guilty enough.

The truth or scientific validity of an interpretation has been shown to be quite unrelated to its power. False interpretations work just as well as accurate ones, whether delivered by a skilled strategic therapist early in brief therapy, or by a classical psychoanalyst after years of concentrated analytic work.[9] The power is in the genuine placebo effect generated by a sanctioned healer's interacting with a sufferer who believes that the healer has the "it" which he or she so desperately needs. After years of such reframing it was second nature for me to come up with an interpretation which I figured Marty would accept. My intervention would be a combination of symptom prescription and exercise therapy. Here's how it went.

I told Marty that although the situation he was in seemed unique, it wasn't such an unusual one, and that while it felt to him that there was no way out of it, I had worked with people with very similar problems, people who had worked hard in psychotherapy and felt a whole lot better in only a matter of a few weeks. Depression, I said, has a way of always tricking us into thinking it will never end, but a depression such as his always does. I am convinced that hope is fundamental in treatment.

I went on to say that he seemed to me to be someone who was ready to give up his old, unsuccessful ways of trying to deal with the problem, someone who was motivated enough to try something new. I told him that I could give him a prescription for some daily programs which had brought previous patients remarkably quick relief from depression, but I added that these were rather difficult assignments which would require an hour of hard work each day. I suggested that perhaps he would like a week to think about whether he was ready to undertake so much effort and whether he had the discipline and fortitude to stick with it. Withholding or delaying a prescription adds power.

"I don't need to think about it," he said. "I'll try anything. It's not just me. It's my kids, my job. The whole works is on the line."

Prescribing the Symptom

I paused before the critical reframing. Then I told him that it seemed to me that, without meaning to, he had been his own worst enemy during the past six months by trying to keep his guilt inside, and that his guilt had been signaling the problem by persistently leaking out and ruining his concentration on everything else in his life.

Marty interrupted with a measured tone. "You're not going to tell me that I should feel guilty more of the time?"

"No," I answered. "You and I both know that you don't need any help with that. I'm saying a couple of things. The first is that I agree with you. I know that you do feel deeply responsible and guilty. The other is that you have got to stop trying not to feel guilty. We both know that hasn't worked. What I am suggesting is that by trying to keep all that pain inside over these many months, you've made it next to impossible for yourself to feel normal again. I figure at some point you're going to have to let your guilt out, and that you might want to get to it reasonably soon before your life gets much worse. There is a way, but perhaps you aren't ready. Maybe you'd like to think about it."

"So what are you suggesting?" Again the measured tone.

"Are you sure you want to go on with this today?" I asked.

"Positive."

I went on. "I've found that what seems to work best in situations like this is to actually schedule the guilt. Sometimes concentrating on our guilt for only a single hour each day can free us up to concentrate on other things the rest of the time. But I should warn you that it's very difficult to think of nothing but our guilt for even a single hour."

"You've got to be kidding," said Marty.

Prescribing Exercise

I went on. "The second thing is that I strongly recommend that you to begin to exercise. My suggestion would be for you to come home from work and leave your kids in day care. Change into sweats and running shoes. Since you live in a rural area and we have plenty of daylight this time of year, I would suggest that you do a solid hour of very fast walking each evening. I want you to walk away from your house for 30 minutes, then walk back home again as fast as you possibly can. As the days go by, you will probably find that you will be covering more and more distance. If you feel like eventually throwing in some periods of jogging or running, go ahead. The trick is to exercise for one hour at a brisk pace, but not to overextend or hurt yourself. It's important that you do these walks by yourself."

"That doesn't sound so hard, but why by myself?" he asked.

"This is the hard part," I said, "the part you might have trouble carrying out. I want you think of nothing but your guilt during that hour of exercise each day. You must force yourself to think of nothing but all of the reasons that you feel guilty."

"Doesn't sound hard to me. All I ever do is feel guilty. I can't stop doing it."

"I can see why it might seem like an easy assignment, but my experience with people such as you tells me that it will be harder than you can imagine." I let that sink in, pausing for emphasis, then went on. "By the way, all is not lost if you can't manage it. If you can just manage to do the exercise alone, it will give you some relief from your depression. It will also get you started working off the weight you've put on during the past six months. But understand this, Marty: if you want to move out of a life which is ruled by guilt, you are going to have to do everything you can possibly do to concentrate on your guilt during that exercise hour each day. It's got to be purged."

Before he left that first day, I told him that I believed his assurances that he was in good health, but that just to be on the safe side I would like to talk with his primary-care physician about his treatment history, his medication, and whether a graduated walk-jog program would constitute any health risk for him. Marty signed the necessary release, which I sent off to his physician along with a letter telling him to expect a call. I told Marty that he should limit his daily assignment to brisk walking for three days, and that unless he had heard from me at the end of that time, he could assume that his physician had seen no problem in gradually introducing jogging into his exercise hours.

The Second Session

A week later Marty returned for his second session. He was definitely not the apathetic, exhausted man who had slumped into my chair the week before. He sat down and made immediate solid eye contact with me. He looked irritated.

"It's not working," he said flatly. Sounded like a challenge. He was angry. I knew full well what wasn't working, but I asked what the problem was.

"It's impossible," he retorted. "The exercise is no problem. As a matter of fact, I'm starting to like it. I can't wait to get home to do it. I'm already jogging maybe half the time, but how in the hell do you expect me to concentrate on nothing but how guilty I am for a solid hour? Its impossible."

"Are you really trying?" I asked with concern.

"Are you kidding me?" he fired back. "Of course I'm trying. Its just plain impossible."

I shook my head and told him that I was sorry to hear that. I suggested that perhaps he was allowing himself to be distracted too easily. I then went on to say that if he genuinely wanted to get better, and if therapy was going to be of any use to him, he would have to try much harder. I suggested putting a rubber band around one of his wrists during his exercise hour and snapping himself each time he found his mind wandering away from thinking about all of the reasons that he should feel guilty.

He volunteered that he was becoming angry with me. I replied that that was a common reaction from people to whom I had given a similar assignment and that his anger at me was a good sign that he was doing the best he could, and that he trusted me enough to express his anger. He softened and told me that he really did want to get well. He promised to try even more diligently to feel guilty during the coming week's walk-runs but couldn't promise how successful he might be.

Session Three

The following week he was steaming when he stormed into my office. He hadn't even taken a chair when he opened with, "Are you sure you know what in the hell you are doing?"

I thought to myself that therapy was proceeding splendidly but inquired what seemed to be the problem.

"You're the problem. You're asking me to do something that's impossible, and you must know it if you have any brains at all. The more I run, the madder I get. Every time I go out, I get madder and madder. I wonder where in the hell you got your degree." He paused, then went on, "For the first time in my life, I think I know what it is to feel genuine rage. When I think of how I set myself aside all these years and tried to keep Jane happy . . . and her screwing around the whole time . . . I've never been so damned mad! I've had fantasies of killing the woman!"

I listened patiently until his feelings gradually subsided. He told me that his work was going better. He was more able to concentrate and hadn't missed a day since he began therapy. He also figured that he had lost a couple of pounds. Before he left I reminded him to continue to work hard at purging his guilt during the week's runs. He gave me a long, silent look before he walked out.

Session Four

Our fourth session was different from those which had preceded. The word guilt was never mentioned. Nor was it mentioned in any subsequent sessions. Marty walked in and opened with, "I am not convinced that you know what you are doing, but I want to talk about my kids."

Marty's life had turned a corner. From being an exhausted and nearly hopeless victim, this man was telling me that he was beginning to take charge of his life. He was asking for input on just exactly what he could do to begin responsibly parenting his children. He was moving the focus from himself and onto to the two boys. We spent that hour and the following one exchanging information and coming up with workable strategies and plans. Marty mentioned that he had played golf with a friend the weekend before.

I saw Marty a total of eight times over the course of several months. I left the door open should he ever want to return for more help. Months later I received a Christmas card from him saying things were good, the kids were healing, and thank you. A couple years later a new patient slumped into my office chair looking pretty bad. He said his friend Marty figured I could help.

Case Review

So what exactly happened with Marty? He appeared to change both dramatically and quickly, and the changes were also durable.

First of all, it is important to keep in mind that Marty was an ideal candidate for psychotherapy. My assessment was that he did not present an immediate suicidal risk. However, he was so very desperate and so very miserable that he was willing to risk new ways of behaving, feeling, and thinking. Change must be fueled by powerful emotions. The word *crisis* in Chinese is made up of two separate symbols, the first representing "danger" and the second "opportunity."

With Marty I was also able to use two of the most powerful tools at my command, symptom prescription and exercise therapy. The first of the two quickly drove a definitive wedge into Marty's uncontrolled obsessive ruminations. The second worked to provide quick relief from his depression. Symptom prescription obviously cannot be used on all depressed individuals, but it is highly powerful for obsessive symptoms, and it seemed like a workable prescription for Marty.

Marty's symptomatic rumination became an even greater ordeal when he attempted to consciously feel nothing but guilt for an hour each day. In addition to making the symptom even more unbearable, perhaps at some level Marty began to realize that this symptom, which for so long had seemed involuntary, actually was something over which he had control. He might also have begun to see the paradoxical humor in our conversations during our early sessions when he was passionately telling me that it was impossible to feel guilty for a whole hour each day, and I was arguing that he was never going to get well unless he did so. After all, the man came in because he couldn't stop feeling guilty. Perhaps all of these things were involved, but whatever the case they were never discussed. If Marty ever realized the volitional or humorous elements in the treatment we shall never know. I would never be so discourteous as to inquire whether or not he was conscious of these things or imply that I had much to do with his rapid recovery. Better that he accept the credit for taking the prescription and trying to follow it, even if it didn't really work and even though I might not have appeared to know exactly what I was doing. Symptom prescription is a very paradoxical and puzzling phenomenon which always tends to "unbalance" patients.

The walk-jog prescription, of course, had a power of its own. It's highly possible that the euphoria-producing beta endorphins and the powerful antidepressant neurotransmitter norepinephrine were more active in his brain both during and for many hours after his daily exercise periods. The fact that he stopped taking his prescription antidepressants after a few weeks of treatment suggests that his jogging might have elevated the activity of endogenous antidepressant neurotransmitters so that the imipramine was no longer required. Substituting exercise for imipramine allowed Marty to function better on the job (the drug is sedating) and also allowed him to begin to lose weight (antidepressants commonly cause weight gains).

The tranquilizing effect of Marty's increasingly intense evening-exercise periods must also have played a part in his being able to set aside the prescription tranquilizers he had been using for months. He had been using Valium for sleep each night, but the drug has a substantial half-life and had contributed to his groggy and lethargic condition at work.

This case is of special interest because the two prescriptions appeared to have a substantial interaction effect. I often prescribe exercise for anxious and depressed patients, and I almost routinely employ symptom prescription for patients who are troubled with obsessions. It is somewhat unusual to work with someone for whom both prescriptions are appropriate. Guilt rumination and strenuous exercise mixed together may create a special sort of chemistry which has significant therapeutic implications.

Marty moved very rapidly from brisk walking, to jogging about half the time, and on to running for an entire hour each evening. He said that the bursts of running felt good and seemed to happen without any conscious effort, that he was increasingly powered by emerging feelings. When I quizzed him about this, it seemed clear that it was anger which had come bursting into his consciousness to fuel his running. The physiological state of running appeared to facilitate awareness of his long-repressed anger.

Guilt may be next to impossible to experience in a body which is highly energized and activated. Guilt is a passive sort of state, associated with deep sighs, shallow and infrequent breathing, a sluggish heartbeat, low blood pressure, and a listless, deenergized state. How can we feel guilt when our heart is pounding, our blood is surging, and our muscles and lungs are working near capacity? These sorts of physiological changes are more closely related to the emotion of anger.

It's commonly thought that guilt is a manifestation of anger turned inward onto ourselves, and Marty's testimony suggests that perhaps the prescription of guilt in conjunction with running has the potential to help us to externalize our anger. Marty discovered that he was not only mad at me but surprised to discover that he had been carrying around a vast amount of anger at Jane. It had been suppressed and largely experienced as guilt because of Jane's final angry act. It seems highly possible that the physiological feeling state of running made it more likely that he would retrieve memories of the times he had felt anger toward her and would build on or intensify those feelings and memories. It also seems likely that such retrieval and intensification would, in turn, fuel his brisk walking and move him toward increased bursts of jogging and running.

The professional literature on exercise and mood is replete with consistent findings that hostility is reduced following exercise. It makes sense that exercise could "put us in touch" with and help us "work out" our anger. While exercise stands as a solid prescription for many kinds of depression, it might be especially powerful when we are dealing with certain people who are both depressed and troubled by pathological guilt.

While exercise can almost universally be applied to depressed individuals, I would like again to underline the fact that symptom prescription cannot. One does not tell a suicidal person to feel more guilty. Symptom prescription, however, is not an issue with most depressed patients. The primary issue is to sell them on the idea of beginning to exercise, and to present it in such a manner that they are likely to both give it a try and keep on doing it.

The Exercise Prescription

In my work with depressed patients I introduce the idea of exercise very early, usually during our first session. I suggest that patients have the resources to dramatically reduce their misery on their own. I point out that it has been scientifically demonstrated that regular exercise reduces depression in most people very effectively. I go on to explain that the exercise need not be intense and that only a few hours a week are required. I talk about how people who began to exercise at a moderate intensity for as little as a half hour three times a week were able to reduce their depression. I add that exercising five times a week has an even more powerful antidepressant effect.

I attempt to emphasize four fundamental points. The first is that *exercise will help*. I am able to communicate this to patients with real conviction and in a very matter-of-fact way since I both respect the scientific literature on the topic and personally believe it, having watched exercise do the job with patients, friends, and myself. Pointing out that exercise therapy has been scientifically shown to effectively reduce depression, and that it has physiological effects which may parallel those of antidepressant and tranquilizing drugs, enhances the power of the prescription for many patients.

The second point I want patients to hear is that *exercise reduces depression quickly*. Here again I emphasize research findings and experience with previous patients. I matter-of-factly state that the patient will feel better immediately after each session of exercise, and that with regular exercise he or she could be symptom-free in as few as three to five weeks.

The third thing I want to get across is the notion of *moderation and flexibility*. The prescription is most likely to fail if it requires too much too soon and is very rigid with regard to schedule or kind of exercise.

Finally, and most important, I stress the point that *the patient has the resources to independently find relief from the symptoms of depression*.

Tailoring the Prescription to Individuals

I always inquire about the patient's current physical activities (usually there is no regular exercise) and ask about what sorts of physical activities the patient used to enjoy in the past. If the patient has or had a *preferred activity*, I will try to build on that activity as the central prescription. It is usually easier for a patient to return to tennis, cycling, basketball, aerobic dance, hiking, or whatever he or she used to enjoy than to begin a new activity which may or may not fit the patient's needs. *Season, facilities, convenience,* and other factors can also have an important part in prescribing an activity that is likely to stick.

People differ dramatically with regard to their capacity to tolerate *boredom*. Some thrive on predictable routines while others cannot tolerate them. For the latter, I suggest a variety of activities. Someone might, for example, go to aerobic dance classes three times a week and go for a long hike or bicycle ride on the weekend. Someone else might go back to playing league volleyball one night a week, jog three times a week, or sometimes lift weights, swim, or play racquetball instead of jogging.

Since exercise can do so much more than simply reduce the symptoms of depression, I always attempt to take *each individual's problems and needs* into account when prescribing exercise in order to increase the odds that the patient will continue to exercise.

For example, a depressed and highly stressed middle-level business executive who works in an environment which constantly provokes pressure and anxiety may get a different prescription from that recommended for his depressed and severely overweight fellow employee who works alone within the windowless confines of the company packaging room.

Since these two depressed patients are middle-aged and remarkably unfit, I would attempt to prescribe a minimum of three periods of aerobic exercise a week—exercise of a sufficient intensity and duration not only to impact their depression, but also to begin to build the sort of cardiorespiratory fitness that would give them some protection from heart attacks and slow the progression of atherosclerosis. I would spell out all of these things to them to help sell the prescription.

I would be especially interested in reducing the resting heart rate and blood pressure in the highly stressed executive. I would encourage him to exercise during his lunch hour. A brief brisk walk could do the job. This midday workout would allow him to work off the morning's accumulated tensions, and perhaps partially immunize him for the afternoon shift. I would also suggest that he park his car (or get off the train or bus) a mile or two from work in the morning and walk briskly to work, reducing his morning anxiety. The evening walk back to his car would serve to impact whatever anxiety he carried with him when work ended.

My special concerns for the overweight packaging room employee would be somewhat different. I would supplement his three aerobic sessions with some long and sustained periods of exercise to work on his weight problem. A later chapter will explain that weight control hinges importantly on our capacity to burn fat as a fuel, and that this whole complex process is best facilitated through long periods of moderate activity. The supplemental prescription for the packaging man, then, would be long walks or bicycle rides several times a week. He might walk for an hour after work a couple of times a week and take a long hike or bicycle ride on the weekend.

Thus, the two patients will be given a common prescription to deal with their depression and their common need for increased cardiorespiratory fitness, but each will be given specific supplemental prescriptions to deal with their unique needs concerning stress and weight control. Becoming informed about the many specific benefits of different forms of exercise allows the professional to confidently make these sorts of individually tailored exercise prescriptions. Wanting and expecting to become less depressed can be sufficiently strong motives for some of us to undertake an exercise program, but the added knowledge that if we exercise in certain ways, we can also significantly impact other important problems can add to our motivation to get started and keep going.

The *social factor* is a very important element in the exercise prescription, since it has to do both with how other people can contribute to our stress and with how they might affect the odds of our both beginning and continuing with an exercise program. Our overstressed business executive may react to most people who approach him on the job with at least moderate apprehension, wondering what sort of demands or problems they are going to present. For him time alone would seem to be very important. A solitary walk or workout at lunchtime might make more sense than a workout with other people, where expectations and demands might override the distraction which games can provide.

The solitary, bored, and overweight patient in the packaging room, however, may require a very different sort of prescription if exercise is likely to take hold. Adult league softball or volleyball might be particularly rewarding and self-perpetuating because of its social benefits. A mixed aerobic program of calisthenics, at the YMCA or at a fitness center, would add a social element during those periods when he was exercising for cardiorespiratory fitness. I would also suggest that he find a friend or family member who might also like to lose weight and get in shape to accompany him on the long walks that are so crucial for him. Thus some of us need time alone for relief from the pressures and demands of others, while others of us require the presence of others to carry out an exercise program which we might not be able to manage if left totally on our own.

A decade ago, when I first began to run, about the only people I met along the byways and streets were other solitary male runners. That has changed dramatically during the past few years. Now it is more common to meet cyclists and walkers, and it is rare to see them exercising by themselves. Bicyclists come in pairs or in groups. I frequently see the same husband and wife pairs on my daily runs, and the groups of cyclists I encounter increasingly include women. The walkers I meet are more commonly pairs or groups of women who probably live along the routes I run. Sometimes I meet a group of three or four young mothers with baby strollers. Whatever the case, they seem always to be striding along rapidly and engaged in animated conversation.

No one can convince me that having someone to talk to isn't an important motivating factor for many people who exercise. Even when I do my weekend-long runs up on the mountain trails, I increasingly run into pairs of women energetically striding along. Predictably, we all seem to be paying only limited attention to the waterfalls, redwood trees, and scattered families of blacktail deer. My concern is with where each footfall will land, since I have already had all of the sprained ankles I could wish for in a lifetime. But the walkers are often very busy talking and making eye contact with one another. I suspect that the brisk walk might sweep away some of the inhibitions which normally are in place, for they talk with speed, feeling, and great energy. In all of my years on the trails and roadways, I have never seen depressed walkers.

I remember some years ago getting a letter from a runner who was in his 70s and retired. His wife had died a few years earlier and one of his eventual adjustments to living alone was to move to an apartment adjacent to a community college. He worked out on the college track late each afternoon when the facility was most populated. There was always someone who was running at his pace, and he loved to run and chat with the students. I suspect that the students must have learned a lot about life while working out with this lean and well-conditioned role model, but he pointed out to me that running with them kept him young by keeping his brain churning with new ideas and new ways of looking at things. He suggested that more older people consider the rewards of settling in next to a college and taking part in classes and various other activities.

One of the best ways to help many people begin and stay with an exercise program is to make the prescription a social one. I always recommend that such people find someone else with similar needs and make a regular commitment to exercise with that person. For the severely depressed patient it is almost imperative that family members or friends be brought into the treatment scheme as exercise therapists.

Therapists Who Walk and Talk

The therapist can make a substantial impact on the life of the patient and can enhance the probability of making an exercise prescription take hold by exercising with patients during their regular psychotherapy sessions. This has a number of payoffs for both therapist and patient. For the therapist the payoffs range from reduced weight, depressed mood, and lower back pain to increased energy and effectiveness as a therapeutic agent. It might also help immunize the therapist from burnout. I run every morning and don't personally need to exercise with patients, but I enjoy walking briskly with patients who are depressed. What's more, I believe that the walking facilitates greater productivity from the patients.

The California psychiatrist Dr. Thaddeus Kostrubala[8] and University of Nebraska exercise physiologist Dr. Wesley Sime[11] have both spent countless hours running with patients, and both of them testify that therapy is somehow more powerful when it is combined with exercise. Sime has pointed out that while most psychiatrists verbalize the benefits of exercise, very few incorporate it into therapy. He has worked as an exercise therapist in conjunction with psychologists and psychiatrists who themselves don't exercise with patients. They refer very depressed individuals to Sime for walk-run therapy. These are patients who may be too anxious either to join a group program or to start to exercise on their own. Sime argues that it is preferable for the therapist who is actually doing the clinical treatment to do the exercise therapy directly, rather than have information transmitted secondhand from the running therapist.

Sime also points out that depressed individuals with whom he runs are often resistant and unwilling to acknowledge that they are making progress or feeling better. For this reason he suggests that depression sometimes feels to him like a *communication disease* which can affect and frustrate the therapist. Psychotherapists know very well what he is speaking about. Day after day we are faced with patients who feel helpless and are victimized by symptoms of all sorts—patients who are experts at using those symptoms to victimize other significant people in their lives, including their psychotherapists. We can all feel defeated, helpless, and frustrated when communicating with a depressed individual.

The psychotherapist who walks and runs with depressed patients and is experiencing exercise's acute mood-elevating effects during the therapeutic hour is going to be more immune to the patient's unconscious manipulative tactics. The therapist who walks with a patient during therapeutic sessions is also likely to have more to offer the patient who is scheduled for the *next hour*. The therapist's mood will be elevated and he or she will be more centered, energized, and relaxed.

While walking or running with a patient might have direct positive effects upon the therapist, there are also potential payoffs for the patient. Both Sime and Kostrubala suggest that the cathartic effects of the patient's physical exertion carry over into psychological catharsis. It makes sense that a trained clinician be on the scene when this sort of rich and highly charged material comes bursting forth during a session of exercise. The presence of a trusted psychotherapist might further facilitate the patient who, feeling as though he or she is in safe and skilled hands, can let it all out.

My experiences parallel those reported by Kostrubala and Sime. Even brisk walking on the part of unconditioned patients seems to "loosen them up." They become less inhibited and constrained and more in touch with their immediate feelings and experience. They become energized and seem more inclined to move to talking about their own needs and what they genuinely feel (rather than what they should feel). I experience them as becoming less self-conscious (concerned about what others might think of their behavior) and more conscious of themselves.

Patients who are walking as briskly as possible seem much more likely to get in touch with their anger and assertive needs—a move in the direction of health for people who typically repress their anger and defer their needs to those of others. My experience is that strenuous running may be even more effective. Perhaps it's just that well-conditioned people have to work harder to "lose their heads and come to their senses" as Dr. Fritz Perls, the founder of Gestalt therapy, used to say. Whether I am running with patients, casual friends, good friends, or strangers I happen to meet at the trailhead parking lot, people seem to become more open, direct, and emotional after they get a couple of miles up the mountain.

There is no research that I know of to back up these notions. The research which has been conducted on the efficacy of exercise as an antidepressant agent is always set up in such a way that talking about problems is prohibited while the individual patient is walking or running along with an exercise therapist. Such research also normally does not involve groups of patients for precisely the same reason. If talk about problems and verbal catharsis had been permitted in such research, we could not have discovered whether or not exercise was an effective therapeutic agent in and of itself.

Future research will have to determine whether exercise in conjunction with psychotherapy is as powerful as or more powerful than the combined effects of the two of them administered separately. But at this early stage, it may be unwise to ignore the input from those few therapists who have had considerable experience running with patients, therapists who consistently suggest that the combination of the two appears to be particularly effective.

If therapists are going to engage in exercise with patients during regular therapy sessions, it makes sense that walking or jogging would be the logical choice. Walking can be easily engaged in while talking, and most therapists can walk out of their offices and find either a park, a mall, or a street where it is possible to walk and talk with patients. Walking or jogging requires no special equipment beyond decent shoes, and these activities can be done in almost any sort of weather short of a hurricane or blizzard. Getting sweaty may be a problem for some of us who aren't comfortable with it and don't have a shower handy. Scheduling a walk-talk session as the final session of the day is one possibility. Another is to schedule such a session as the final one of the morning, if the noon hour allows the therapist to have access to a shower.

I have also found that patients can handle seeing their therapist dressed informally in sweats, and for that matter even seeing their therapist sweaty. Professional stature does not seem to suffer. Some patients comment that they like experiencing the therapist in this altered role. It makes them feel that we are making a special effort and that we are human.

Another strategy is available for professionals who work in conjunction with other therapists in either private or public clinics or agencies, places where there is a large pool of patients for whom exercise would be an effective prescription. It is also an option for the more isolated private practitioner who has a reasonably large practice. It's not difficult to organize walk-run sessions for pairs or groups of depressed patients. Getting two or more people together to exercise three or four times a week in the absence of the therapist(s) offers the possibility of enhanced compliance for the patients as well as the probability of some effective peer therapy and support. Another option for the therapist is to meet with a group of depressed patients once a week for a two-hour walk-talk group therapy session. When both therapist and patient(s) exercise together, potential benefits may be magnified. The therapist has the opportunity to see how individuals actually do interact with others rather than hearing "unconfirmed reports" during weekly individual therapy sessions. Kostrubala engaged in running therapy with groups of patients who had a variety of diagnoses such as schizophrenia and anorexia nervosa.[8]

Summing up, there are all sorts of ways that exercise might be used to make both psychotherapy and psychotherapists potentially more effective. The therapist who prescribes exercise may be of significantly greater help to depressed patients by helping them dramatically and quickly reduce depression without resorting to the use of antidepressant medications. Informed prescription of exercise can also impact other problems which impact the patient's physical and mental health. The therapist who exercises with patients may significantly speed up the important affective-cognitive aspects of the therapeutic process by introducing a condition (exercise) which facilitates patient catharsis, and by being there on the scene to deal with it. The therapist who exercises with patients also is likely to be more immune to the power of the patient's symptoms, and is going to reap personal benefits such as elevated mood, reduced tension, and increased energy which will make him or her more effective with other patients, and which will facilitate personal survival in a profession where burnout is a serious problem.

Patients Who Resist the Exercise Prescription

Some patients who could benefit from the exercise prescription are very resistant, listing all sorts of reasons why it is impossible or impractical. Let's suppose a patient has rejected even walking with the therapist or a family member in order to relieve the symptoms of depression. One possibility is that the depression has a payoff.

All symptoms bring us misery, but they can also give us the power to make our world more predictable as well as to control our important relationships. Depression can regulate nearly all aspects of an individual's family life. In adults, for example, a depression can regulate things such as arguments, sex, conversation, attention, caretaking, and social activity. It can set all sorts of limits on what the children are allowed to do, things such as being noisy, having friends in, or having the TV or radio blaring. If an individual's depression appears to fall in that category—miserable to the suffering patient, but worth it in terms of the many payoffs and the degree of interpersonal control that it affords—it makes sense that the patient would resist any efforts to let it go.

It's well to remember that for such a patient this whole process is largely unconscious. Awareness of personally using a symptom such as depression to manipulate our loved ones would be unacceptable. We wouldn't want to see ourselves as the sort of person who is so easily threatened and so inadequate that we must deal with our inadequacies in such underhanded ways. Besides, we didn't choose to be depressed. It happened to us.

Sometimes a depression begins for very understandable reasons but continues long beyond what would normally be expected for reasons that don't appear to make sense. When the patient's depression is hanging on because of the social control and payoffs it affords, I utilize the patient's resistance to change.

During the first therapy session I almost invariably introduce the possibility of exercise with depressed patients. I am very cautious about how I present this, since it is partly a responsible presentation of treatment-relevant information and partly a probe to measure resistance. If the patient resists beginning any sort of individual exercise, I will ask whether we might walk together during our sessions, or I will ask if there is a friend or family member we could enlist to walk with the patient on other days. It is important to tread carefully in such circumstances, doing what is possible to motivate the reluctant patient or providing social support for the patient who needs it in order to get started, but being very careful not to push an exercise prescription onto a clearly resistant patient whose symptoms might be hanging on because of secondary gains.

When I sense resistance in a patient, I immediately stop suggesting exercise, to avoid having to contend with "yes, but" resistive responses. I accept what the patient offers—an unwillingess to exercise—and attempt to reframe it so that the patient's resistance might be used against his or her depression.

The reframing for the resistant patient is usually centered on readiness. I speculate out loud that the patient clearly is not ready to begin to exercise. Perhaps the patient needs to be depressed longer or even to become more depressed in order to generate the motivation to do something about the depression. Clearly the patient is not now miserable enough. Perhaps, even though the patient says that he or she wants to be rid of the depression, life has become somehow easier or more comfortable with depression as a constant companion. Maybe we should begin to focus on how we can better adjust our lives around the depression.

Work with the patient's family can speed things up by breaking patterns of behavior which are generated in response to the symptomatic depression. If the therapist gets the family members to agree that predictable ways in which they have been reacting to the patient's depression have not worked, they may be willing to try new ways of behaving which will take the payoff away from the symptom. If the depression no longer regulates and controls the behavior of the patient's family, it can usually be terminated with dispatch.

Different Forms of Depression

So for what kinds of depressed patients can we prescribe exercise? It would actually be far simpler to address the question of when and why exercise is inappropriate, since exercise seems to be at least an appropriate adjunctive prescription for almost all depressed individuals who are not at some sort of health risk.

I know of no research which deals with exercise as a treatment for bipolar patients. Such disorders are so clearly biogenically predisposed and respond so specifically to biochemical treatment that exercise seems like an unlikely candidate at this juncture. If, as suggested in an earlier chapter, mania is related to excessive adrenergic neural activity, exercise could conceivably worsen manic symptoms. On the other hand, a bipolar patient in a depressed phase might benefit from exercise since it's highly probable that exercise elevates levels of norepinephrine.

Dr. Egil Martinsen has shown us that even hospitalized and medicated patients with a history of many major depressive episodes will not only accept the prescription of exercise but benefit significantly more from a combination of exercise and traditional biochemical and psychotherapeutic treatments than from the traditional therapies alone. A major depression is a very serious and debilitating depression, so Martinson's work is very significant.

Each year 60,000 to 100,000 Americans receive electroconvulsive therapy. In light of Martinsen's findings, it would be worthwhile to see whether individuals who are being cared for at home or are living in institutions because of depression so severe that ECT appears to be the only alternative could and would respond to exercise therapy. Could highly supportive, one-to-one exercise therapy, in conjunction with antidepressant medication, reduce symptoms sufficiently to make ECT and its side effects unnecessary? Likewise, if an individual has received ECT, could exercise alone or exercise in conjunction with antidepressant medication significantly reduce the recurrence of depressive episodes. Martinsen's work suggests that these might be viable treatment options, and such treatments might yield benefits beyond simply the avoidance of electroconvulsive therapy's negative side effects. A substantial one is that trained technicians, volunteers, family members, relatives, or close friends could all contribute to the treatment program. Besides the obvious cost-effectiveness, there is the potential for other social psychotherapeutic benefits.

Many investigators have consistently shown that exercise is a powerful, rapid, and durable treatment for depressions of lesser severity. Such depressions have variable causes, and exercise can serve very nicely as an adjunct to psychotherapy for some, and as a primary treatment for others where psychotherapy is not required.

The research which has so consistently demonstrated that exercise reduces depression has encompassed men and women from high school to retirement age. While there has been little work as yet on children, my guess is that we have nothing to lose by prescribing exercise for depressed kids. If depression has isolated a child, I would suggest making the exercise prescription a social and supportive one. We cannot be sure, but the odds are that exercise will elevate depressed moods in children in a manner similar to that consistently observed in adults. We are only beginning to realize what a pervasive problem depression is among our children, since it is so often obscured by other more obvious symptoms. The prescription of exercise for depressed children is a research project waiting to happen.

Biochemical Imbalances

Those of us who suffer long periods of depression for which there are no significant environmental or psychological causes (dysthymia) are very likely suffering from a biochemical systemic imbalance, a condition which might ordinarily be treated with antidepressant medication. There is the possibility that regular exercise could correct an aminergic deficiency as effectively as antidepressant drugs, and with beneficent rather than unwanted side effects.

Exercise may counteract the depression caused by the buildup of melatonin levels in our brains when we experience a lack of sunlight during winter in extreme latitudes (seasonal affective disorder or SAD). I observed residents of Oslo, Norway, seeking every moment of daylight and available ray of January sun by getting outdoors to walk and cross-country ski. Being outdoors and exercising is a well-established pattern of life for these people who dwell just below the Arctic Circle, and it may very well be that their high activity levels compensate for the months they endure seeing little or nothing of the sun. That Vikings would go mad in the winter if they could not exercise seems to be a cultural truism. Four-thousand-year-old rock carvings of skiers have been found in the north of Norway.

Here in the United States the SAD susceptibility line runs roughly from Boston out to San Francisco. People who live above that line are increasingly at risk for winter's depressions. Bipolar individuals have been found to be particularly sensitive to changes in sunlight, but many of us can react rather dramatically to decreased sunlight. Some salespeople get depressed when they visit San Francisco during a foggy period.

The solution for those of us who suffer from seasonal affective disorder is to try to spend an hour in the sun each day, either outdoors or in front of a sun-facing large window. Greater relief may be found by combining physical activity with sunlight. Aerobic exercise in front of a sun-facing window or an hour's activity outdoors would be ideal ways to combat this sort of depression.

In northern latitudes where there is only darkness for months on end, the solution is to spend time (reading, writing, or eating meals) in the presence of artificial light. Full-spectrum (Vita-Lite) light bulbs, which reproduce outdoor daylight and are used for growing indoor plants, were originally used to treat SAD. But it appears that diffuse light of any sort which is of sufficient intensity (it should match the level of outdoor light shortly after sunrise or before sunset) will do. Fluorescent bulbs are often used with a diffusing screen. The amount of time required in the presence of the artificial light varies from individual to individual, but usually about five days of treatment will effectively reduce SAD symptoms. Where there is no electricity, chopping firewood and walking may have to do.

Normal Uncomplicated Grief

While it is unlikely that any grief is completely "uncomplicated" (by psychological factors), some kinds of grief are far less complicated than others and do not ordinarily require the attention of a psychotherapist. The depression associated with grief can be expected to strongly ebb and flow for a year or more, and exercise can be an effective tool to help us get through the grieving period. My experience is that there are people who are better equipped than psychotherapists to help with the psychological aspects of treatment and support for the individual who is suffering from uncomplicated grief.

A 35-year-old woman who was a student in my exercise-and-mental-health class one fall is a case in point. About 10 months prior to beginning the class both her husband and son had died violently. When the shock reaction wore off, she became quite dysfunctional and had pretty much retreated to the isolated sanctuary of a small cottage. Fortunately, she made contact with the Center for Living with Dying, a United Way organization made up largely of volunteers who had dealt with the loss of people whom they loved. A volunteer from the organization began to call on Sarah. The volunteer got her up on her feet and walking, at first only partway down the block and back, but as time went by, eventually all the way to the grocery store. Before too long Sarah began to drive to the center for group meetings.

She found a kind of understanding among the people in her group that she simply could not have found in any other circumstance. The volunteer who was selected for her was a woman who had also lost most of her family in a single tragic event. She could offer the most authentic sort of understanding, and all of the people at the center were living testimony that it was possible to survive the loss of loved ones and get past the disabling depressions which result when such losses occur. What's more, the support and understanding which the people at the center had to offer were free, so that their gifts were both genuine and precious.

The volunteer who got Sarah to walk more each day knew well the healing power of activating deeply depressed people and was keenly aware that they frequently didn't have the resources to do it alone in the dreadful aftermath of loss.

Signing up for university classes was a big step for Sarah, and she didn't know whether she could concentrate well enough to pull it off. As the semester wore on, she became more social and began to make friends. A couple of times she showed up for class in sweats, lugging a tennis racquet along with her books. Her mood seemed to be changing for the better. I saw her sometimes joking with friends, in contrast to the serious conversations I had observed early on. A few weeks prior to the end of the semester she told me that she had been running daily for almost three weeks and that she had not only got through the anniversary of her loss but was feeling less depressed than in years. She smiled and asked, "Why didn't someone tell me about this running sooner?"

For Sarah, the volunteers from the Center for Living with Dying provided all that she needed. She recently told me that she now feels strong enough to volunteer at the center to pass on the gifts of understanding and support which she received.

For many of us, uncomplicated grief does not require professional help, and unless we are at some sort of risk, all of us who are grieving can benefit from exercise. It is important to remember that many of us do not have the resources to get started on our own and will need support and help at first. Going for daily walks with a friend who has lost a loved one one can help her or him turn the corner. It is also important to remember that grief does not occur only when a loved one dies. When anyone leaves us permanently, we grieve. Exercise can help us get through the depressions arising from a love affair gone sour, a separation, a divorce, or any nest suddenly left empty. Talking with others who have been through a similar loss is the other sensible way to take care of ourselves.

Besides grief there are other reasonably uncomplicated circumstances where we sometimes must simply bear with long-term unavoidable stress. Illness and disability in a family member or long-term unresolvable difficulties on a job which we cannot afford to leave are examples of the sorts of sustained stress which can eventually result in depression. Exercise can help us through these tough times.

When Psychotherapy Can Help

There are, of course, all kinds of depressions which are seriously complicated by unresolved psychological issues. The loss of a loved one through death, divorce, or separation can certainly be complicated. Professional help can be invaluable in working through unresolved issues or in helping to examine both personal and interactive factors involved in the breakup of a relationship.

There are a whole host of psychological disorders whose symptoms cause us repeated difficulties in interpersonal relationships. For example, the symptoms associated with the various personality disorders tend to isolate us and erode our self-esteem. Many of our depressions result from the stress and hopelessness produced by our repeated maladaptive behaviors. When this is the case, the routine use of regular exercise by itself can be unwise in that the symptom relief which it provides allows us to avoid seeking professional help to rid ourselves of the maladaptive behavior patterns which lie at the root of such depressions. If such a self-generated depression is severe, exercise can be prescribed by the therapist as an adjunctive therapy to provide symptom relief while the primary psychotherapeutic treatment takes place. The therapist's exercising with the patient might further speed up the process.

Prescribing Exercise for Our Own Depression

Before directly addressing the question of just exactly how each of us can self-prescribe exercise to impact our own moods, it is important that we have more information concerning exercise's other important physiological and psychological effects. For example, if we want to use exercise to treat our depression, it would be helpful to know how we might best design a program which would also have significant effects on our other concerns with things such as weight, anxiety, or cardiovascular fitness. It is also important for us to know what risks are associated with exercise, so chapters on these topics will precede the chapter which deals with self-prescription. Let's move now to a consideration of exercise and anxiety disorders.

Chapter 8

Exercise, Anxiety, and Phobias

Exercise can play a significant role in the treatment of phobic disorders. I will introduce this chapter with two cases which involve phobias, one a case of simple phobia, and the other a case where a panic attack resulted in agoraphobia. These cases serve to illustrate several things. First, they make it clear that phobias have different causes and may require different treatments. One case will illustrate how exercise therapy can serve as an adjunct to long-term interpersonal psychotherapy, substituting for tranquilizing medication to reduce the symptomatic anxiety which interferes with so many facets of daily functioning. The second case will demonstrate how exercise can be utilized in behavior therapy to provide effective short-term treatment for agoraphobia.

Jill: A Case Study

It was one of those splendid October days. A brilliant blue sky, a soft warm sun, and crisp autumn air which carried both pungent reminders of summer and hints of the coming winter—the sort of day that made me want to hoot and holler about the magnificence of simply being alive.

I'd just returned to the counseling center, fresh from a couple of hours of doubles volleyball out under the huge elms which had filtered benign sunlight down onto our playground. I couldn't have felt better when I walked into the waiting room to introduce myself to a new patient. Her intake form told me that she was a freshman, 19 years old, and that she had asked to see someone at once. Jill followed me back to my office, where she sat down and very shortly began to tremble and shake. When she stopped sobbing, raised her head, and was finally able to speak, her first words were, "I think I am going crazy."

Jill was both ashamed of and bewildered by the dramatic appearance of a frightening and disabling disorder. A few nights before she had gone on a first date with Jim, a young man from her dormitory. She had gradually befriended Jim during the early weeks of the fall semester and had spent increasing amounts of time with him. She trusted him. On their first formal date the two of them went to a movie together. Partway through the film Jim turned toward Jill and smiled, at the same time reaching over to take her hand. She screamed, bolted upright, and stumbled out of the theater. When Jim caught up with her, she was sobbing, apologetic, and embarrassed. She felt that she had humiliated him, but could offer only apologies since she had no explanation for what had happened. When Jim reached out to comfort her, she jumped backward out of reach.

As days passed, things went from bad to worse. She found that she was very uncomfortable when any men were physically close to her. If she felt she might be touched, she panicked. Her life was dramatically altered. Going to classes became difficult, and it became difficult to concentrate on lectures and reading assignments. She was almost constantly obsessed with her phobic reaction to men. It made absolutely no sense to her, and the only explanation she could come up with was that she was going insane. It was this fear that brought her to me.

My main concern that first day was to let her know that what she was experiencing was not an unusual phenomenon. I explained that such irrational fears were called phobias, and that the panic attack which had seemed to set off the phobia and the phobia itself were most common problems. I also explained that phobias frequently appear with dramatic suddenness and often don't seem to have any immediate apparent cause. But I underlined the fact that phobias always have causes, that with time we would both find out what the causes of her phobia were, and added that phobias respond well to psychotherapy.

Jill felt relieved and a whole lot better as the hour progressed and this knowledge sunk in. Demystification, support, and hope are powerful interventions for someone who is suddenly overwhelmed with strong feelings and strange behaviors which make no sense. I cautioned her that she might have to live with her fear for some time, that it could require months to get to the bottom of things and put an end to her irrational fears. I pointed out that it was unwise to move too quickly with these kinds of problems, and that we had to come up with strategies to help her function while we worked together on getting to the bottom of her problem.

We discussed ways to minimize the risks of setting off future panic attacks, practical ways to avoid putting herself in potentially threatening situations. We also talked about what to do if she unavoidably found herself in a threatening circumstance: to immediately, but very slowly and deliberately, walk away from the situation as soon as she began to feel uncomfortable. I suggested that she might think about telling Jim about her visit with me, so that their friendship could continue to develop without his unknowingly threatening her. If she felt that her fearful behavior required explanations to others, we decided that she might consider telling them that she was being treated for some problems having to do with fears of physical contact.

I also told her that she could ameliorate her anxiety and get through this difficult time by beginning to engage in some sort of regular physical activity. I suggested very brisk walking as she moved about campus, to and from her dormitory and from class to class. We talked about what sorts of exercise she enjoyed; weighed in the factors of convenience, daylight hours, and safety; and decided that daily evening swims in the women's indoor campus pool could help relax her for study and sleep.

The combination of weekly therapy sessions, minimizing threatening social situations, speaking directly but briefly about her problems when necessary, and daily exercise made it possible for her to function adequately and survive academically. She was able to concentrate sufficiently well to take lecture notes, read her texts, pass exams, and sleep without our having to resort to the use of drugs.

It was during a session early the following May when Jill's adolescent traumas came bursting forth into consciousness. All the missing gaps were filled in a single hour. Her story involved a long period of sexual abuse and her father's eventual suicide. The enormous outpouring of repressed memories and feelings that spring day had immediate significant consequences. While Jill and I had considerable work to do sorting out and dealing with all of her feelings about both of her parents, her phobic reaction to men dramatically diminished and shortly ended. Certainly both the upwelling of the repressed material and the dramatic end to the phobia were the common results of the seven months of psychotherapy which had preceded, a relationship which gradually provided the platform of trust and security which made it safe for Jill to remember.

There were no shortcuts to Jill's treatment. Directly attempting to remove her symptoms would have been unwise indeed, what with the indications of repressed trauma. She required long-term attention to heal and to learn to trust again.

Phobias respond well to psychotherapy; behavior therapy techniques are most commonly employed. For many years "systematic desensitization" prevailed, but "flooding" now seems to be the preferred method. It's quicker and cheaper. In both cases the patient is exposed to the feared object or circumstance, either gradually through fantasy and imagination during a state of deep physical relaxation in the therapist's office, in the case of systematic desensitization, or suddenly and dramatically in the company of the therapist out in the real world when flooding is utilized. People cannot rid themselves of phobic responses without exposure to the feared object, and contemporary behavior-therapy methods are not unlike the old prepsychotherapy solutions for the simple phobias which had clear, uncomplicated precipitating circumstances. The historical cure for a phobic reaction to horses (after being thrown), for example, was to get back on. No way could you avoid the anxiety. You had to face it, live through it, and keep getting on the horse until it was gone or at least reduced to a level of uneasiness which could be lived with.

Jill's case makes it very clear that not all phobias can be safely addressed by simply quickly removing the symptom—getting back on the horse. The case also suggests that exercise can sometimes be used adjunctively as a substitute for tranquilizing and sedative drugs. Most phobias are far less complicated than Jill's, and many of them can be addressed more quickly and directly by somehow getting the patient back on the horse and dislodging the anxiety which is associated with whatever the patient's particular horse might be. Exercise can play a very important role in behavior therapy as applied to phobias.

It was the British psychologist Arnold Orwin who reasoned that exercise might be a powerful tool to use in the treatment of phobias.[8,9] He pointed out that the "physiology of conversion" which characterizes religious practices in some primitive cultures often involves drumming, dancing, and chanting to the point of exhaustion. This physiological state of exhaustion appears to facilitate relief from sin, evil, and the anxieties associated with them.

The state of physical exhaustion became central in the highly effective technique which Orwin developed for the treatment of both simple phobias and agoraphobia. It combines some of the features of both systematic desensitization and flooding, but it offers several special advantages. This example from my own practice illustrates how it works.

Jennifer: A Case Study

Jennifer's husband, Al, got off work early in order to bring her to my office for her first visit. Their lives had seemed relatively uncomplicated and normal until Jennifer had suffered a panic attack while shopping alone one day in a department store which was located within a large enclosed suburban shopping-mall. Jennifer had never had a panic attack before. This terrifying experience developed into agoraphobia. She was deeply fearful of being alone in public places, where she might have another panic attack and be without help. Her anxiety-free space had slowly collapsed to where she now spent most of her time at home. She no longer drove or went anywhere without Jim or her close woman friend who lived next door. Life for Al and Jennifer became complicated, with commonplace daily activities now requiring great care and planning. Jill's agoraphobia appeared to be the product of an unfortunate first panic attack which happened in the wrong place at the wrong time. Both she and Al seemed sincerely to want to be rid of it.

I talked with the two of them about how common panic attacks and resultant phobias are, especially for women, and how amenable such phobias are to treatment. I specifically outlined the process which probably occurred as Jennifer's phobia took shape and helped them to understand how anxiety played a central role in her problem. I went on to explain that physical exercise was one of the most potent antianxiety forces available, and that it would play a central role in Jennifer's treatment. I predicted that, if both of them would participate in the treatment, we could very likely be rid of the phobia in a very short time. Needless to say, they were both glad to hear that and were eager to get started. I made the usual arrangement to consult with Jennifer's physician in order to make sure it was safe for her to walk and run, and I asked them both to meet me for our second session at a convenient shopping center which had an enormous parking lot. The three of us were all to wear sweats and running shoes. Jennifer had no problems with shopping centers as long as she was accompanied by someone she trusted.

A week later the three of us met one morning in the shopping center's nearly empty parking area. We sought out a distant unoccupied area which was devoid of traffic. Our goal that morning, I explained, was to experiment with just exactly how far Jennifer had to run at a brisk pace in order to bring on a state of marked breathlessness which would last for several minutes. While we checked out distances and the length of breathlessness after each run, I talked to them about treatment.

Specifically I asked Al to begin to spend some time working with Jennifer each evening at home. I was concerned that she begin to do something about the discomfort she felt about leaving home by herself. I asked Al to stand in front of their home while Jennifer ran rapidly as far down the street as was necessary for her to feel breathless. She was then to continue to walk away during the few minutes required for her to catch her breath. She was to turn around and walk or slowly jog back to him the moment she felt the first twinges of anxiety. They were to repeat the sequence at least three times each evening after Al came home from work and were to expect that Jennifer would gradually increase the distance she could run as her fitness improved. Jennifer was to meet me back in the parking lot in a week, once again in sweats.

Jennifer's assignment that week went something like this. Having established just how far she could run to produce a few minutes of breathlessness, we measured off that distance from the entrance to the mall to a point where I stood with her in the parking area. She was to run from where I stood to the entrance, where she would arrive acutely breathless. I assured her that the physical exhaustion she felt would prevent a panic attack. She was then to walk around the entrance catching her breath until she first began to feel hints of anxiety, at which point she was to walk or jog easily back to me. On her fourth and final trip of the day Jennifer surprised me by walking through the mall door moments after she arrived. She stayed perhaps a half minute before coming out and walking around a while and then jogging back to me.

Jennifer continued to do her prescribed running at home on a daily basis. Her runs there became longer and consumed increasing time. Then she began to do her runs alone in the afternoon before Al came home. Apart from expanding her anxiety-free space, she was beginning to enjoy the running and looked forward to the tranquil feelings which always followed. During our third session at the mall, Jennifer took to walking alone inside the mall during the minutes when she was catching her breath. The time she spent inside increased with each successive run. Before the last run of the day I suggested that she consciously attempt to panic and faint upon entering the mall, and I bet that she couldn't manage it. She laughed and refused the wager. Anytime patients can smile or joke about their symptoms or problems, things are looking good. Jennifer and I spent another hour at the mall a week later, extending the time she spent alone inside. Then there was no longer a need for therapy. I received a Christmas card from the two of them that year telling me that Jennifer seemed permanently free of her problem and that they were getting along fine.

Exercise Therapy for Phobias: Theory and Strengths

Orwin has trained nursing staff, spouses, and welfare officers to provide "running therapy" for patients who suffer from agoraphobia or simple phobias. He has used running therapy successfully to treat more than 100 patients who were hospitalized with agoraphobia and other disorders. Some patients ran toward feared stimuli or circumstances, and others ran away from safe, anxiety-free havens. The number of treatment sessions required varied with the duration and intensity of the patient's symptoms and the degree to which the symptoms possessed secondary psychosocial gains.

Orwin points out that this form of treatment offers a number of unique strengths which allow it to significantly impact the anxiety associated with phobic disorders. The first is that the instinctive response to anxiety (to walk or run away in retreat) is used to control it. Another important factor is that the ongoing autonomic-nervous-system excitation caused by the vigorous physical activity competes with and inhibits the anxiety reaction and allows the patient to be aware of the normally fearful environment without the feeling of fear. The sympathetic branch of the autonomic (self-governing) nervous system is responsible for the "fight-or-flight" reponse when our bodies are mobilized by stress (such as running). The therapist can assure patients that when they arrive at the vicinity of the feared stimuli in a state of breathless exhaustion, they will not experience anxiety. While there are common features in the two physiological arousal states, there are also important differences, and patients cannot experience the two states simultaneously. Finally, there is an important cognitive component. The physical state produced by running not only competes with anxiety, but further allows patients to redefine or find a sensible explanation for the emotional arousal. If any autonomic component of the anxiety reaction is experienced, it would be cognitively labeled as a part of the body's response to physical exercise.

There are, in addition, some very pragmatic advantages to this form of treatment for phobic disorders. The main one is that the spouse, another family member, or a technician can be quickly instructed to administer the treatment. It follows that such treatment would be very cost-effective. Both of these are important considerations in a society where anxiety disorders are the most common group of psychiatric problems.

Treatment Problems with Phobias

Happy endings are not always the case with phobic individuals. Sometimes the phobia is very resistant to treatment of any kind, or if it is relieved by therapy, it quickly recurs. When these things happen, a number of different factors might be involved.

The first is that the patient may be strongly biochemically predisposed to the panic attacks which persistently regenerate and fuel the agoraphobia. Women are far more subject to panic attacks than are men, and some women are much more susceptible than others, a finding which suggests biochemical predisposition. Minimizing stress, especially during premenstrual periods, may help, but medication for the panic disorder might also be required. The minor tranquilizer alprazolam (Xanax) and the tricyclic antidepressant imipramine (Tofranil) are the drugs most commonly prescribed. These drugs serve to minimize the likelihood of panic reactions. With such drugs, the agoraphobic individual can spend time in feared situations (crowded stores, elevators, away from the safety of home, and so on) without the usual anxiety reaction. This sometimes allows deconditioning to take place, so that when the medication is reduced and terminated, there is a possibility that the old avoidance and anxious reactions to those circumstances will be minimized to the point where they no longer control the patient's life.

If a phobia does not respond to treatment, another possibility is that the phobia has such important secondary gains that the patient needs it in order to importantly control his or her interpersonal relationships. In such cases the patient and the patient's spouse may need the symptom to restore or maintain balance in an unstable relationship. Marriage partners frequently unconsciously triangulate a third factor into a threatened relationship to hold things together rather than directly face up to what is troubling the two of them.

Some married couples settle in for the long haul with agoraphobia as an uneasy but unconsciously welcome third partner. The symptom somehow stabilizes the relationship or makes it possible for the marriage, however unbalanced, to work. Such partners often talk about doing something about the problem, but the payoffs for both husband and wife are significant enough for each of them so that they never actually act on their avowed intentions. However unbalanced the newly defined roles which result from making agoraphobia a full-time family member, those new roles might somehow be only a modest exaggeration of what both of them privately needed but could not publicly admit. He, for example, might privately or unconsciously want a wife who stays at home, never socializes, and mothers him with the sort of caretaking he never received. She might similarly be satisfying unconscious dependency needs.

In other couples a phobia may recur after treatment because of important ongoing and unresolved marital problems. The secondary gains may be satisfying to the patient but may be frustrating and unacceptable to the spouse. Removing the symptom with therapy may result in a recurrence, but it may also precipitate discussion of what is really troublesome in the relationship. The couple moves from the uneasy surface calm which prevails when spouses speak to one another metaphorically (with the symptom and related behaviors) to the tempest of speaking directly about one another's needs and feelings. Removing the symptom can sometimes make discussion of the real issues more likely and can speed up the process of psychotherapy.

Normal Anxiety and Exercise

A large number of cross-sectional studies spanning many decades consistently reveal that people who exercise with regularity (endurance athletes such as distance runners, rowers, and wrestlers) consistently report experiencing less tension when at rest than those of us who are the same age, but sedentary. The most logical place to seek an explanation for such reduced tension would be in exercise-induced physiological changes.

Exercise produces a very widespread and objectively measurable physiological relaxation response. Walking, jogging, and cycling at mild to moderate intensities have all been shown to reduce physical tension, and symptom relief is especially pronounced among individuals who are clinically anxious. However, relief predictably occurs for all of us, regardless of our resting tension level. The relaxation effects are measurable in the brain (increased hemispheric synchronization), in the dorsal spine (as reflected in certain reflex tests), and in skeletal muscles (in decreased spindle activity as measured by an electromyograph). Because the same effects can be produced through heating either the brain stem or the entire body, University of Southern California professor Dr. Herbert de Vries[4] has suggested that one strong possibility is that the acute relaxation response produced by exercise is probably the result of the higher body temperatures which it produces. The typical jogger we see moving along the roadside has a core temperature of around 103 degrees Fahrenheit.

University of Michigan physiologist Dr. Joseph Cannon[3] points out that our bodies respond to strenuous exercise in precisely the same manner that they do when invaded by bacteria or viruses. The release of pyrogens (endogenous leucocyte mediators) results in reductions of zinc and iron concentrations in our blood, an increase in leucocytes (white blood cells), and an increase in body temperature (a fever). The body becomes a lousy place for germs to live. They get fried and eaten. Another effect is that our bodies become very relaxed—as after a long sauna or a dip in a hot tub.

This pyrogenic response may partially explain why many individuals who exercise consistently, but who don't overdo it to the point of exhaustion, report never having had a cold or the flu since they began regularly engaging in endurance activity. What they more typically report is that they sometimes seem to "begin to come down with something" but that it rarely turns into a full-fledged cold or case of influenza. The typical week or 10-day illness is avoided.

When I first began to run at the age of 50, like so many other people I was almost consumed by the many rewards which it bestowed. I went overboard for a few years until I grudgingly learned to accept moderation. At the very beginning I was amazed to discover that I had the hidden resources and courage to do things which my rational brain had always contended were impossible. I ran (struggled through and somehow survived) my first marathon only six months after I first took up running, and during the next year I ran five more of them. Crazy behavior.

I gradually tapered off running those 26.2-mile races and moved to racing shorter distances. Many years later I pretty much stopped racing altogether. I settled into running four or five miles a day at a very comfortable pace. I still went to the mountains on weekends for the longer journeys which gave me the sort of hit that my weekday runs couldn't fully provide, but I moved into a phase where I was running simply for physical and mental health.

When I was exercising excessively, racing actively, and doing so very many marathons, I was constantly ill and injured. I had to give up all exercise for six months at one point because I refused to give a plantar foot injury time to heal. I picked up each influenza and cold bug that passed my way. I was especially prone to illness when I was peaking for a marathon and straining against my speed and weekly mileage limits. I was constantly reminded that for me, the difference between being in peak shape and being in a state of exhaustion (with lowered resistance) could be small indeed. When I run 30 to 40 miles a week at a modest pace I never injure myself from overtraining, and I have only passing hints of illness which announce their arrival, but seem never to develop into anything.

My experience of consistent moderate exercise and an end to most colds and influenzas is one which many people report. While these sorts of reports, at this point, lack scientific backing, it makes sense that a daily fever plus a flood of germ-fighting white blood cells may reduce the probability of becoming ill when our bodies are invaded by various pathogens. Of course, this can all be erased by overtraining to a point where resistance is constantly or periodically at a low level.

Exercise and Muscle Relaxation

The muscle relaxation which follows exercise is quite impressive, and muscular tension is one of the common physiological measures of the anxiety tension state. Dr. de Vries has done a number of studies which have consistently demonstrated that exercise can significantly reduce electrical activity or tension in muscles.[4] What is so encouraging about his findings is that this sort of significant physiological tranquilizing effect holds for normal and clinically anxious men and women of both sexes and has been demonstrated in young adults as well as in middle-aged and elderly men and women. Even better news is that the tranquilizing effect results from even brief periods of very moderate exercise and that it is measurable for at least an hour and a half after exercise ends.

In one experiment de Vries compared four random groups of 10 elderly people who believed they suffered from anxiety or tension problems. One group walked at a very moderate pace (producing a heart rate of only 100 beats a minute), another group received 400 mg of the tranquilizing drug meprobamate (Miltown), a third group received 400 mg of lactose (a placebo), and one group served as a control (no treatment). The exercise treatment was significantly superior to all others (which failed to differ from one another) in the reduction of electrical activity in the subject's muscles. De Vries suggests that moderate exercise might be used as an alternative to tranquilizing drugs in the treatment of the normal anxiety which we periodically experience. The advantages include immediate self-prescription, convenience, affordability, and beneficent rather than unwanted side effects.

This very widespread general-relaxation response, which impacts both our central and peripheral nervous systems, may in part constitute the basis of what runners refer to as "the high." It may add to or interact with the effects of beta endorphin (which is also released up to 10 times the normal level when we run a fever), indolamine (serotonin), and the catecholamines (norepinephrine and dopamine) to form a biochemical platform for healthy exercise dependency. It's apparent that as exercise experience accrues, this postrun afterglow becomes increasingly central as a motive to sustain regular workouts. Runners go out and train when they don't feel like it, and they persist even when the first mile or two feel lousy, because of the guaranteed afterglow which they know will follow.

Psychological Measures of Anxiety

State Anxiety

Besides objective physiological methods for assessing tension, there are simple psychological tests to measure how much anxiety we are experiencing at a given moment (state anxiety) and to measure our typical baseline anxiety level (trait anxiety). The State-

Trait Anxiety Inventory (STAI)[10] has been widely used in research to determine whether exercise can impact the anxiety which we experience and report. There is now an impressive body of research which shows that exercise can predictably reduce state anxiety, but that light exercise such as walking may not be effective.[7] Somewhat more vigorous activity, such as running or its aerobic equivalent (70 to 80 percent of $Vo_{2_{MAX}}$), appears to be necessary to reduce psychological state anxiety. Dr. Robert Brown at the University of Virginia has been measuring the psychological effects of exercise on students for more than a decade, and at this point he has data on more than 5000 students who consistently showed reductions in anxiety following exercise.[2] But, as in the case of depression, exercise is not the only variable which has the power to reduce state anxiety.

In a classic experiment at the University of Wisconsin, state anxiety was assessed in 75 adult men who were then randomly assigned to one of three different treatment groups.[1] One group exercised for 20 minutes at 70 percent of their $Vo_{2_{MAX}}$. Another 25 men were assigned to a group which engaged in meditation, and the final 25 rested quietly in a sound-filtered room for 20 minutes. These latter "time-out" subjects were monitored for heart rate, oxygen consumption, and skin temperature in order to control for the effects of attention. Posttreatment state-anxiety scores were significantly lower for both the exercise and meditation groups. However, the time-out group also showed reduced state anxiety after 20 minutes of quiet rest, and the change in their anxiety scores did not differ from the results found for the exercise and meditation groups. These sorts of findings have caused Morgan[1] to speculate that perhaps any sort of distraction from anxiety-provoking thoughts and stressful stimuli can bring about the reduction of state anxiety. He has pointed out, however, that there are data which suggest that the effects of exercise may last longer than those of other distractors.

Exercise, such as jogging, is associated with reduced state anxiety for from two to four hours in individuals who have low to high levels of anxiety. Whether or not exercise itself causes the reduced anxiety, the effect is very predictable and has been consistently demonstrated in both laboratory and natural settings.

Trait Anxiety

Two of my Norwegian friends, Dr. Kari Fasting and graduate student Hilde Grønningsæter, from the National College of Sports went to Denmark a few years ago and collaborated with scientists at the University of Odense to study the effect of physical activity on unemployed adults.[6] They knew that the best single predictor of mental health during unemployment was whether a person felt his or her time was occupied, and that unemployed people tend to become physicially inactive. They were particularly interested in finding out whether regular exercise could lower trait anxiety in these individuals. Earlier research on trait anxiety (one's typical baseline level of psychologically experienced anxiety) suggested that after prolonged training (months) the level either does not change at all or, less frequently, decreases. Earlier research had also suggested that decreases in trait anxiety were more likely to occur in individuals who were both clinically anxious and in poor physical condition.

Sixty-four unemployed Danes, aged 24 to 45 were matched for age and sex and divided into three groups. One group exercised with either calisthenics, volleyball, or badminton, always followed by swimming twice a week for two hours. People in this group were allowed to choose how much of each of the three kinds of exercise they wanted each day. Kari Fasting told me one day that this sort of freedom of choice and flexibility was very important in keeping the participants exercising. A placebo group (who had social interaction and attention) met during the same time and engaged in the discussion of various topics led by a social worker. The third group received no attention and served as a control. A variety of psychological measures as well as an oxygen uptake test were given before and after the three-month experimental period.

The results were quite interesting. For one thing, both the exercise and control groups showed significant increases in oxygen uptake at the end of the research period. The increase was more significant in the exercise group, but the increase in the control group was also significant. Postexperiment interviews confirmed that many of the men and women in the control group had begun to exercise on their own, a finding suggesting that exercise may be a viable means of coping with the stresses of unemployment, one which some people seek out on their own. While there was a negative correlation between trait anxiety and fitness, it was not a significant one.

The other findings of interest were that the exercise group showed significant reductions in trait anxiety over the three-month period, and that within that group the change was manifested only in those individuals who had had high trait anxiety when the experiment began. The low-trait-anxiety people in the exercise group showed no change over the course of the three months.

Trait anxiety is very difficult to assess, as tests are always somewhat contaminated by various other personality traits and by real-life stressors which occur at the time of testing. These difficulties may account for the mixed experimental findings by those who have investigated the impact of exercise on trait anxiety. The mixed findings might also be partially the result of doing research with people who represent a broad range of resting anxiety. While most experiments show no change in trait anxiety in response to exercise, those that do show a change in a positive direction suggest that people with clinically high trait anxiety as well as those in poor physical condition might benefit most from regular exercise over the course of many months.

Exercise appears to be a viable intervention for dealing with the acute episodes of anxiety which intermittently occur in all of our lives. Research has consistently shown that even brief exercise at very moderate intensities in adults of all ages significantly reduces physical tension, and that somewhat more intense exercise reliably reduces psychological state anxiety. These findings suggest that those of us who live sedentary lives and work at sedentary jobs may suffer from unnaturally high levels of anxiety and tension, the partial consequence of a lifestyle which is at odds with a physiology designed to function normally with regular physical activity.

Exercise and Panic Attacks

Because intravenous injections of sodium *dl*-lactate can induce panic attacks in individuals who have a high susceptibility to such attacks, and because exercise has been shown to elevate blood lactate levels dramatically, highly anxious people who are subject to panic attacks have been frequently cautioned not to exercise strenuously. However, there appear to be no cases of exercise-induced panic attacks. Exercise at intensities which elevate blood lactate levels up to 10 times resting levels have failed to produce panic attacks in either normal or highly anxious individuals.[5]

Apparently, injected buffered lactate does not have the same effects as our endogenously produced lactic acid. The metabolic routes and the behavioral effects are quite different. Exercise appears to be a safe prescription for anxiety, even for those of us predisposed to high levels of anxiety and panic attacks.

Research Summary

A review of recent research concerning the effect of exercise therapy on anxiety permits considerable optimism. Whether or not exercise per se reduces anxiety, it is consistently associated with lowered psychological state anxiety as well as reduced physiological tension in both normal individuals and those of us who are chronically anxious. Exercise is a safe and viable prescription for reducing state anxiety for men and women of all ages who are not at physical risk. The tranquilizing effects of exercise are acute, lasting for from two to four hours. There is also the possibility that regular endurance training may lower our baseline level of trait anxiety, especially if we are clinically anxious and physically out of shape. Mild to moderate exercise produces a predictable general physiological relaxation-response whose peripheral effects on skeletal muscle tension are more powerful than those of a minor tranquilizer. Finally, when used within the behavior therapy framework described by Orwin, exercise can play a significant role in the rapid treatment of simple phobias and agoraphobia. Small effort, big payoff.

Another View of Anxiety

Anxiety has a bad reputation. Like mosquitoes, gophers, and other pests or inconveniences, it is something professionals and laypeople alike typically try get rid of. But anxiety is a normal and important part of our lives and, like nearly everything else, has both beneficial and negative sides.

Dr. Carl Jung pointed out that fire has the capacity to both destroy and create (it can destroy a house or forge steel). He suggested that the fires within human beings are emotions, and that they, too, can both destroy and create. Anxiety does, of course, fuel psychopathology (agoraphobia is a good example), but Jung reminded us that anxiety also has the power to destroy (maladaptive defensive behaviors) and to fuel positive change (new ways of feeling, thinking, and being).

Most therapists would concur that personality change is not possible without experiencing anxiety, and that anxiety is a necessary and powerful force in psychotherapy. Optimal anxiety in a new patient should not be so high as to cause him or her to become dysfunctional (speechless and overwhelmed with emotion, or motivated to flee the session) but should be high enough to allow the therapist to observe and assess ego strength, defenses, and coping mechanisms.

Existential-humanistic psychotherapists have embraced anxiety as a necessary and positive force in human change. Like Jung, they conceive of anxiety as a clarion summons, a important signal which alerts us to avoided opportunities for living, chances passed by, potential unrealized, and risks not taken. For them anxiety might sometimes be not the cause, but the consequence of poor existence or living.

Jung cautioned against unthinkingly or indiscriminately medicating away anxiety and depression, the very states which might be necessary for personal change. Tranquilizing and antidepressant drugs can be effective tools which enhance healing, but they can also be temporary solutions which perpetuate the causes of our misery and make healing impossible.

The central point here is that we must use caution when we deal with a patient's anxiety or, for that matter, our own. Just as we can unwisely reduce anxiety through the use of drugs, so too can we unwisely reduce it with exercise. Compulsive exercise which effectively keeps pathological anxiety tolerable is maladaptive if it prevents the psychotherapy which may remove the cause of the anxiety. On the other hand, when appropriate, exercise can be a marvelous adjunctive treatment device for dealing with a number of anxiety disorders, and is the perfect prescription for the normal anxieties which are so much a part of our daily lives.

Chapter 9
Other Psychological Outcomes

A man's stride betrays whether he has found his own way. . .
I love to run swiftly.
And though there are swamps and thick melancholy on earth,
Whoever has light feet runs even over mud
And dances as on swept ice.

—Friedrich Nietzsche

When we consider the many biochemical and physiological components of anxiety and depression, it makes sense that these conditions might be the disorders most affected by exercise therapy. The many biochemical and other physiological consequences of exercise would suggest that it might also have application in the treatment of other disorders where there are very significant physiological components. The personality, adjustment, and classically "neurotic" disorders, which are the common focus of psychotherapy, are not likely candidates unless these disorders also result in the symptomatic depression or anxiety where exercise can be adjunctively utilized. However, substance abuse disorders and cognitive losses associated with aging in normal individuals are more logical candidates for exercise interventions. The self-mastery aspects of exercise therapy would also suggest that it might have a role in dealing with improving our self-esteem.

While the possibilities are many, research on exercise therapy's other psychological outcomes is, for the most part, scattered and preliminary. This chapter touches on some of this research. It concerns both normal individuals and those with mental disorders.

Self-Concept and Self-Esteem

Self-concept and self-esteem have been the focus of a great deal of research. Many researchers have attempted to relate physical fitness and exercise to changes in how we perceive or value ourselves. These studies cover a wide range of the population, including elementary-school, high-school, and college students as well as both adult and elderly men and women. Reviews which span more than a decade have attempted to make sense of this continuing research.[2,13,20,23]

Self-concept is a term which covers a great deal of territory. Its definition usually includes our sense of identity and self-worth and our perceived capabilities and limitations. Self-sufficiency and self-efficacy are also involved in the definition of self-concept. Body image and discrepancies between the real self (how we perceive ourselves) and the ideal self (who we would like to be) also play a role in our self-concept. Finally, the word *self-concept* is often used interchangeably with *self-esteem*.

It's difficult to experimentally isolate self-esteem because it interacts and covaries with so very many other personality variables. It has been shown, for example, that exercise reduces tension and elevates physical self-concept.[36] It has also been shown that both weight training and running elevate self-esteem in women, but that weight training does so more than running, a finding causing one investigator to conclude that weight training also elevates self-sufficiency (which is a component of self-esteem).[35] Thus, self-esteem is a somewhat slippery concept to corral.

One conclusion which seems to emerge from many studies is that *self-esteem is more likely to be elevated when exercise is introduced to special populations.* While studies of exercise and self-esteem done on individuals who make up the general population reveal conflicting results, those done on special groups in which individuals are initially in poor psychological or physical health show exercise to have a consistently positive effect on self-esteem or self-concept.

For example, exercise has been shown to elevate self-concept in obese male teenagers as well as in adult male patients who were being rehabilitated from physical injuries.[9,10] The experiment which demonstrated that self-esteem rose with both running and weight training, but that the increases were greater after lifting weights, is of relevance here. It is of significance that the subjects of the research were women, and who are typically physically less strong than men, and who might be expected to show increased self-esteem with strength training.[35] Another investigator discovered that both young and mature women showed elevations in self-concept after 12 weeks of weight training even though there were no measurable changes in body composition.[5] Another group of women who took part in a physically and psychologically challenging outdoor program of physical activity also raised their self-concepts, although those elevations were gone eight weeks later.[27]

These experiments, which so consistently show increases in self-concept among special groups of individuals suggest that a reduction in the disparity between the real self and the ideal self might play a role, but more importantly, they suggest that the consequences of exercise might have to be related to factors which caused the reduced self-esteem. It makes sense that obese adolescent boys who lose weight through exercise or disabled men who become more self-sufficient as the result of an exercise program would feel greater self-esteem.

Research is very inconsistent with regard to whether exercise has to significantly improve fitness in order for the self-concept to be elevated. Studies where a significant aerobic training effect (increased cardiorespiratory fitness) has been demonstrated typically show increases in self-concept.[13] However, several studies reveal that simply thinking that we are fit or are becoming more fit will do the job as well.[5,18,24] One recent investigation demonstrated that individuals who received passive electronic muscle stimulation and those who took part in a combined aerobic-nonaerobic exercise program both elevated their self-concepts and lowered their anxiety.[4]

It appears that activities which enhance our self-sufficiency, reduce the discrepancy between our perceived and ideal selves, focus positive attention on ourselves, alter our body image positively, or increase our perceived fitness may all raise our self-esteem. Research findings are contradictory, and it appears that experimentally elevated self-esteem may often be short-lived. One thread of consistency which seems to run through these many studies would suggest that if we wish to elevate our self-esteem, the causes of our low self-esteem simply cannot be ignored when designing effective treatment strategies.

This would seem to be particularly true when we regard exercise as a treatment tool. For example, if our self-esteem is low because of deficient social skills, no education, or pathological behavior which isolates us from others, it would be asking a great deal from exercise to require that it make things right. If, on the other hand, our low self-esteem has roots in our body image, and is the result of dismal fitness, weight distribution, or obesity, exercise might be just what the doctor ordered. Exercise might positively focus attention on ourselves and the roots of our low self-esteem, reduce the gap between our perceived and ideal selves, and provide us with an increased sense of control and self-sufficiency.

Thus, while exercise can make us feel better by elevating our mood and reducing our anxiety, *its effectiveness in enhancing our self-esteem and making such changes last may hinge on whether its consequences are related to the causes of our devalued self-esteem.*

Hostility

While the effectiveness of exercise as a tool for elevating self-esteem appears to hinge on the specific causes of our impaired self-esteem, exercise does have a very predictable general effect on another important personality variable. Anger and hostility are consistently reduced by exercise. Brown[6,7] has been testing students in mental health courses at the University of Virginia for many years, and he now has a data base of more than 5,000 students who demonstrate that regular exercise predictably reduces hostility. Fremont and Craighead[15] found the same thing in research which compared exercise to cognitive psychotherapy. Berger[3] has also demonstrated that exercise has an acute or immediate hostility-reduction effect on both unconditioned and conditioned swimmers. This probably comes as no surprise to parents, who for years have sent angry and unruly children "outside to play." Kids always seem less aggressive when they return from physical play. The same thing is true of adults.

Apart from widespread scientific support, there is evidence of this relationship between exercise and reduced hostility everywhere we look. How many times have we seen boxers and other athletes bloody one another in the fiercest sort of combat, then when the final bell or whistle blows, we see them hug one another with genuine affection and respect? Other things equal, these combatants were undoubtedly easier to live with when they got home as well. The sedentary office worker who comes home with a load of unexpressed hostility after a day of frustrating non-physical work is a very different matter.

A few years ago I received a long letter from a runner who spoke of the relationship between hostility and exercise. He wrote:

> . . . I started running and gave up smoking at age 33 when I began to take over responsibility for my health. I began walking and jogging around a golf course near my home long before the running craze hit us. I noticed that after I exercised, I always felt so much better. It left me with a warm afterglow. I was a very aggressive lacrosse player (even a dirty player), but I found that running left me calm and relaxed without any desire to hurt or even dominate. I just love gentle running. . . .

More to the point is what has happened in our prisons in America. It appears that building recreational facilities and sport programs within prisons has changed these institutions more than any other correctional innovation.[33] Exercise programs have made prison life tolerable for inmates and have made prisons safer places for inmates and guards alike.

Apart from our prisons, crowding thousands of anonymous and sedentary spectators into huge sports stadiums also frequently results in violence. Stadiums are not as safe as they used to be, especially when alcohol is involved. It would be a far better thing for everyone if we were all on the playing fields exercising ourselves rather than in the stands watching others. Working out releases tension and reduces hostility. Not working out allows tension and hostility to build within us and sometimes we explode. People around us are safer if we exercise. Couch potatoes make ominous ticking sounds.

The Young and the Old

We have seen that exercise appears to positively impact self-concept or self-esteem more consistently when it is applied to special populations. The same thing is true when we consider some of the other psychological consequences of exercise. Special groups seem to benefit most.

Normal children, for example, do show improvement with regard to locus of control (a greater sense of personally being in control of themselves rather than being controlled by outside forces) after a program of physical activity.[12] However, the effect of exercise on other important behaviors such as intellectual functioning and academic performance of normal schoolchildren is inconsistent. A review of relevant studies finds no support for the notion that physical activity might enhance intellectual functioning in normal children.[13]

Such is not the case for retarded children and adults. Retarded individuals tend to be more sedentary than the general population, and a review of several studies reveals that exercise has a significant positive effect with regard to intellectual functioning, social skills, and motor proficiency in retarded individuals across a very wide age range.[13]

Exercise seems also to have very significant effects on the aged, another population group which tends to be sedentary. Improvements in intellectual functioning have been associated with exercise programs for normal elderly men and women and for hospitalized geriatric mental patients.[26,31] Dr. K. Walter Schale,[32] who has been studying aging at Pennsylvania State University for more than 30 years, concludes that people who led physically active lives during their middle years do not show significant intellectual capacity loss after age 60. The recent National Institute of Mental Health survey of mental disorders in America found that college graduates showed less intellectual impairment with aging. "Use it or lose it" seems to be the rule.

Dr. Schale prescribes square dancing for elderly people, suggesting that it has aerobic benefits and exercises mental skills as well, since the dancers must remember the caller's movement sequences and convert them to organized motor behavior. These two components are also incorporated in rhythmic aerobics programs which have been developed for elderly or partially disabled individuals who have limited flexibility or must do aerobic routines while seated. It appears that physical training is a viable tool for arresting or reversing some of the physical degeneration which occurs in the aging process.

Psychotic Disorders

There have been a handful of experiments involving exercise with geriatric and adult Veteran's Administration hospital patients suffering from schizophrenia and other psychotic disorders.[8,11,22,30,34] A review of these experiments reveals that they have typically employed very modest exercise intensities which are insufficient to produce cardiovascular conditioning effects, and that the selection of patients for fitness training has also been biased.[13] The behaviors which were measured in these investigations included things such as increased self-care, increased daytime activity, reduced hyperactive behavior, and increased behavior control, as well as responses on a large variety of personality tests. The results of these experiments suggest that there was no change more frequently than there was improvement, but the research itself is so filled with problems that it is impossible to speak with certainty about the effect of exercise on psychotic symptoms.

The California psychiatrist Dr. Thaddeus Kostrubala has treated a number of schizophrenic patients with running therapy and has been amazed at the positive results, reporting that his patients have changed dramatically, becoming less symptomatic and sometimes reducing or discontinuing medication. He sounds a cautionary note by pointing out that these changes could be the result of his own enthusiasm and the extra attention that was paid to these patients. He does not contend that distance running is a cure for schizophrenia but only reports the consistently positive results associated with the small sample of patients with whom he worked.[21]

Substance Abuse and Dependencies

As substance abuse is one of the most common mental disorders in America, one would expect considerable research to have been completed on the efficacy of exercise as a treatment. This unfortunately is not the case. While inpatient treatment programs commonly incorporate exercise, little is known about its effectiveness.

This gap in research is an important one, not just because substance abuse is so prevalent in America, but because, in theory, the important biochemical and physiological components of such disorders make them potential candidates for exercise therapy.

Alcohol Abuse and Dependency

While alcohol use has a long history, the story on exercise as a treatment for this disorder is a rather short one. Research groups have examined the effect of exercise on middle-aged and hospitalized male alcoholics.[14,16,25] These studies reveal very little, as they typically either were poorly controlled or showed only small improvements in functioning in some patients. One study, for example, split 20 hospitalized male alcoholics who had been drinking an average of 18 years into jogging and control groups. The joggers ran one mile each day over the course of 20 days. At the end of that period the joggers showed reduced sleep disturbances while the controls did not.

More recently a Canadian research team enlisted 46 male and 12 female alcoholic patients living in five Quebec treatment facilities to participate in aerobic training (one hour daily, five times a week for six weeks) as an adjunct to their regular multidisciplinary therapy, which included daily group therapy.[29] Those who exercised showed significant fitness gains (decreased heart rate, increased maximum oxygen uptake, and reduced body weight). Ninety days after treatment ended, 69 percent of the exercisers were still dry (about twice the percentage of the control patients who had received all aspects of the treatment except exercise). Among the patients who could be located, the same percentages held after 18 months, but none of the exercisers who were located had maintained their improved fitness. The problem with this kind of study is that "enlisted" patients don't fit into a true experimental framework. We don't know if more of them stayed dry because they volunteered to exercise (were more highly motivated to do whatever was necessary to quit drinking), because of the exercise itself, or both.

What with alcohol dependency being the most common mental disorder of American males, there is an urgent need to explore efficacious treatment programs which will help patients detox and stay dry. The primary chemical agents used in detox are enormous doses of minor tranquilizers such as Valium or Xanax. These drugs impact an important brain system (the benzodiazepine-GABA receptor complex) in a manner similar to alcohol and make the coming down less painful. But patients must reduce the dosages of these drugs and eventually stop using them altogether.

While exercise may not impact the benzodiazepine-GABA receptor complex in our brains, it appears to produce important changes in the central nervous system as well as in many of our peripheral systems. These physiological changes have the potential to produce feelings of euphoria and well-being, but more importantly, they elevate mood, decrease pain sensitivity, and have very significant tranquilizing effects. Future research should explore the potential of exercise as an adjunctive treatment for detox and the maintenance of an alcohol-free life. Exercise might gradually substitute for the decreased dosages of tranquilizers and eventually for the alcohol itself. Such a treatment program would require considerable individual attention since compliance would be a tough issue. But tough or not, America needs to begin to do something about the alcohol abuse and dependency which seem to touch all of us in one way or another.

Other Substance Dependencies

If there is an absence of quality research on exercise and alcohol, the rest of the chemical-dependency landscape is bleak indeed. As in the case of alcohol, exercise is often an integral part of a treatment program for individuals detoxing from the opiates and amphetamines, but there is an absence of experimental data which show that it actually is effective.

Testimony abounds. A substantial number of individuals have reported to me that they had begun to run in order to stop or control smoking or excessive drinking, and that running was central to their being able to stop their addictive behaviors. Surveys have shown that as many as 50 percent of committed nonsmoking runners once smoked. But these sorts of reports fail to prove that these people stopped drinking or smoking as a consequence of beginning to run. People might have stopped smoking, cut back on their drinking, changed their diets, and begun to exercise in response to some other powerful motivation which demanded a lifestyle change. Nonetheless, the potential of exercise as a treatment is worth exploring.

It would seem that exercise has considerable potential for both detox and control of a variety of chemical dependencies, since biochemical and other physiological consequences of exercise seem to parallel the effects of some of the drugs we use and abuse. Research in earlier chapters has shown that exercise is accompanied by increased aminergic (norepinephrine, dopamine, serotonin) and opiate (beta endorphin) activity in the brains of rats, and considerable indirect research suggests that exercise may produce similar neurochemical changes in human brains. Similar changes result when we take addictive drugs.

Nicotine

Our responses to nicotine, for example, include increased norepinephrine and dopamine activity. We get an activating rush of higher blood pressure and increased heart rate followed by a period of tranquility. The response to exercise is nearly identical, except exercise doesn't plug up our arteries, deposit tar in our lungs, or send carbon monoxide and a variety of carcinogens out into our bloodstreams. But the psychological hit, the broad physiological response, and the subsequent tranquility produced by exercise are similar to those produced by nicotine and are in all probability mediated by the same neurotransmitters. A cigarette-mediated hit lasts for about a half hour, but an exercise hit can produce both tranquility and energization for several hours.

The physical stress of exercise may also provide euphoric benefits mediated by beta endorphin. Exercise may have potential as a substitute for nicotine and could have a central role in smoking cessation and control. This is an important area for future research, since even though fewer and fewer Americans are smoking, nicotine dependency still afflicts more than one in four of us and causes smokers to die prematurely from nearly all forms of disease.

Cocaine and Speed

Methamphetamine (speed) and its chemical relative cocaine both dramatically elevate dopamine activity in our brains. Amphetamine floods dopamine brain systems by facilitating excessive dopamine release, blocking reuptake, and inhibiting the enzymes which ordinarily break down or degrade this neurotransmitter. Long-distance truckers, and others of us who have needed to stay awake or remain vigilant, have sometimes used amphetamines. But too much speed or cocaine and we can induce an acute paranoid psychosis. Such a toxic acute psychosis can be promptly terminated by simply stopping the use of the drug which precipitated the psychosis. However, even a single dose of speed causes the degeneration and permanent loss of dopamine cells in our neostriatum, a more recent basal-ganglia brain structure whose function is to generate signals for slow movements such as the sort required for postural adjustments like standing, sitting, and walking. Regular long-term use of speed may produce Parkinsonian symptoms.

While exercise produces impressive dopamine activity, it is not in the same ballpark as speed or cocaine. Drs. Otto Appenzeller and David Schade[1] report that dopamine levels in the peripheral blood elevate to 300 percent above baseline in individuals who are running a marathon, and that these runners get an bigger hit after they stop, when their dopamine levels elevate to as much as six times above normal before beginning to drop back down to normal levels.

There is increasing evidence that cocaine, which is both a stimulant and an anesthetic, produces physical dependency, and both cocaine and methamphetamine produce psychological dependency. The withdrawal symptoms of these two drugs are similar and include at least a short period of depression. Exercise could function as a partial substitute for a dopamine hit and could also elevate moods and aid in tranquilizing patients who are undergoing detox.

The Opiates

A whole variety of street and prescription narcotics such as morphine, codeine, Demerol, Percodan, and Darvon are chemical keys which fit into the same receptor sites as our endogenously produced beta endorphin. The opiates which we inject and ingest also produce the same anesthetic and euphoric effects. If exercise results in increased endorphin activity in our brains (as it does in the brains of rats), it could serve as a viable component in detox and control programs which target heroin and prescription narcotic dependencies.

Substance Abuse Research

Research on exercise treatment and the various biochemical dependencies might not be as difficult to conduct as we assume. Compliance would be the primary problem, and such research would demand a large number of exercise therapists to responsibly monitor and support individual patients while they exercise. The many exercise therapists required to provide such individual attention might be recruited as volunteers from the community. Apart from the general population of individual exercisers, there are bicycle, swimming, running, and walking clubs which might want to make a contribution to such a research-treatment project. Some members of such clubs may be people who have had dependency problems themselves. There are also members of Alcoholics Anonymous and Narcotics Anonymous who exercise regularly. These men and women who work out to help themselves stay clean could be trained to be ideal exercise therapists since they are acquainted with dependency. They can listen, provide support, recognize the usual defensive behaviors of substance abusers, and would have a solid belief in the power of exercise as a stay-clean tool.

Hyperactivity

The dopamine response to exercise suggests that it might be a viable treatment or adjunctive treatment for hyperactive children. The amphetamine drug Ritalin (methylphenidate) is currently the treatment of choice, since it does not have the appetite-suppressant qualities of other amphetamines, and is not likely to retard growth in children. Like exercise, Ritalin elevates dopamine activity but has the curious effect of calming hyperactive children. Dr. W. Mark Shipman, who was medical director of the San Diego Center for Children for a number of years, experimented with exercise as a treatment for hyperactive elemementary-school children.[28] Shipman was able to reduce Ritalin dosages and, in some cases, stop drug treatment altogether in many of the children who took to running on a daily basis. These children appeared to have had "extra medication" on the days when they ran and were much less distractible and more able to maintain attention span in the classroom, especially during the two to four hours which followed running sessions. Their teachers reported that they were less disruptive and more manageable, motivated, and responsive after running.

Autism

Drs. Paul Hardy and Kiyo Kitahara at Boston's New England Medical Center believe that increased endorphin levels may reinforce a feedback loop which can explain self-inflicted pain activities in animals and humans.[19] Head banging, for example, commonly causes injuries in autistic children. These two doctors thought that exercise might provide an alternative source of endorphin release, and they designed a twice-a-day exercise program for a number of autistic children. Their early findings are quite positive.

Summing Up

Exercise appears to have the greatest impact and potential impact on mental disorders which have strong biochemical and physiological components. It may have potential within programs which treat chemical dependencies, but research is lacking in this area.

Special populations, or subgroups, seem to reap benefits from exercise which are not always enjoyed by members of the more general population. Problems concerning self-esteem have been effectively treated with exercise therapy, but the success of such therapy hinges importantly on whether the consequences of exercise relate to the causes of the impaired self-concept. Individuals who are obese, physically weak, or rehabilitating from physical injuries, for example, are good candidates for raising self-esteem through exercise.

Sedentary populations also seem particularly appropriate for and responsive to exercise therapy. While intellectual functioning in normal young people and adults does not improve with exercise, such functioning significantly improves in retarded individuals of all ages, and in aged normal men and women when they begin to exercise.

Let's move on now to a consideration of the physical benefits associated with regular exercise. Those of us who are going to begin to exercise to deal with a depression or with anxiety might want to tailor a program which will also deal with other health concerns.

Chapter 10
The Physiological Outcomes

Dr. William Haskell is a well-known authority on exercise who does research in the Heart Disease Prevention Program at Stanford University's Medical Center. In a recent summary of the many rewards associated with adopting a physically active lifestyle, he points out that in addition to the psychological benefits of reduced depression, anxiety, and hostility, there are a number of other physiological benefits which have varying degrees of scientific backing.[19]

Haskell points out that those which have the greatest scientific basis are how exercise contributes to the maintenance of optimal body weight or composition and the normalization of fat and carbohydrate metabolism. Benefits which have also been reported in some circumstances are prevention of coronary heart disease, reduction of systemic arterial blood pressure, the prevention and alleviation to low back pain syndrome, and maintenance of bone mineral content with aging. He also reports that there are a number of disorders where patients show clinical improvement with exercise: Type I diabetes, chronic obstructive lung disease (emphysema and bronchitis), renal (kidney) failure, and arthritis.

In this chapter we will take a close look at these and other health benefits associated with physical activity. Exercise is said to contribute to both the quality and the quantity of our lives. Let's begin with research on whether exercise might actually add to our years.

Exercise and Longevity

You might argue that some of us who remain physically active and live to be very old were biologically blessed, that this genetic gift predisposes us both to engage in physical activity *and* to live longer than others. While there is certainly some truth to such thinking, it isn't the whole truth. What's more, we can't ethically test out such a notion. We cannot randomly assign thousands of human babies to forced active or sedentary lives and then wait around to see when they die. There is, however, a growing body of epidemiological evidence which strongly argues that exercise *per se* has a protective, life-prolonging effect. Other things being equal, those of us who exercise with regularity will live longer than if we had remained sedentary.

More than 20 years ago the British scientist Dr. Jeremy Morris discovered that London's very physically active double-decker bus conductors had far fewer heart attacks than did the more sedentary men who simply sat and drove the buses—this being true even when confounding factors such as obesity, stress, and hypertension were factored out.[31] Morris also found that other British civil servants who walked to work, and those who played hard when off the job also had fewer heart attacks than those who rode to work and those who avoided strenuous leisure-time play.[32]

This same inverse relationship between exercise and heart attacks holds true even when we compare active people with other even more active individuals whose prodigious activity takes them right off the charts. A research group headed by epidemiologist Dr. Ralph Paffenbarger of Stanford University studied a group of nearly 4000 San Francisco longshoremen for a period of 22 years.[36] These men labored on the docks before the age of labor-saving automation and container cargoes. Paffenbarger split the dock-workers into two groups, those extremely active men who burned 8500 or more kilocalories (kcal; what we ordinarily refer to simply as calories) at work each week and the very active men who burned less than that amount. He found that the group who burned 8500 or more kcal per week on the job had significantly fewer heart attacks than their somewhat less active co-workers. This is quite a significant finding because Paffenbarger did not compare sedentary men with physically active men. He compared very active men with even more active men and still found differences in heart attack rates. We would have to jog 75 or more miles a week to burn off 8500 kcal. The men in the less active group, who burned fewer than 8500 kcal a week, very likely burned off more than twice as many calories each week as do those of us in professional occupations and light trades. This does not suggest that we must all jog 75 miles a week to cut the risks of heart attacks. What it does spell out is that exercise is a very powerful factor in determining the odds of a heart attack.

These longshoremen demonstrated the *specific protective effect of physical activity*. The less active men had twice the rate of heart attacks and three times the rate of sudden-death heart attacks of the more active longshoremen. Thus, activity appears to be specifically related to the risk of heart attacks and is especially related to those which result in sudden death.

This specificity of effect was further revealed when the effects of smoking and hypertension were examined. When the longshoremen were divided into smoking and nonsmoking groups, those who smoked died more frequently from a broad range of heart and circulatory disease, from all forms of cancer, and from lung cancer than did nonsmokers.

When the longshoremen were divided into groups which had above- and below-average systolic blood pressure (the higher of the two blood-pressure figures is generated by ventricular contraction), yet another spectrum of diseases was revealed. The hypertensive longshoremen (whose systolic blood pressure was above the group average) died more frequently from an even broader assortment of heart attacks and strokes as well as from hypertensive heart disease.

This sort of stuff is the raw material of epidemiology. A single such investigation suggests only tentative answers to questions which, for ethical reasons, cannot be put to a true experimental test. But if the results of many epidemiological studies are consistent, they carry great weight. A number of epidemiological studies consistently show the inverse relationship between exercise and mortality for people of all ages and races. These studies are also consistent in demonstrating that the protective effect of exercise is specific. Those of us who remain physically active are less likely to suffer death from coronary disease and a subsequent heart attack than those of us who live more sedentary lives.

But do we all have to become double-decker bus conductors or longshoremen in order to reap the benefits of exercise's protective shield? The best answers to questions about how much of what kind of exercise delivers how much heart attack insurance are found in data from an ongoing epidemiological study of Harvard alumni being conducted by a second research group headed up again by Paffenbarger.[37] A group of 17,000 Harvard male alumni, aged 55 to 74, who entered the university between 1916 and 1950, have provided information on their typical physical-activity levels. Harvard University has provided information about their physical health, their family histories, and the sports activities in which they engaged while they were enrolled as students. Death certificates supply the whens and whys.

The 16th-year report of this continuing study reveals that *almost any sort of physical activity has a role in prolonging life, but that not all kinds of activity provide heart attack protection*. Specifically, walking, stair climbing, light sports activities (bowling, baseball, boating, dancing, and golf), and strenuous sports activities (basketball, running, mountaineering, skiing, tennis, and swimming) were all inversely related to death from all causes. The primary relationship was found to be between exercise and deaths due to cardiovascular and respiratory causes. The exceptions were light sports activities, which influenced deaths from all causes but did not influence the incidence of deaths due to coronary heart disease. This study suggests that protection from heart attacks appears to be provided by walking, stair climbing, and strenuous sports activities, but such protection may not be provided by light exercise such as golf and bowling.

Just how much exercise is necessary to provide a protective effect becomes evident when we examine the number of kilocalories expended each week in the various sorts of physical activities which have been shown to reduce death risk. Before we translate the findings of the Harvard study into kilocalories per week and related risk reduction, here are a couple of rules of thumb which relate to the number of calories we typically expend in familiar activities.

Most of us who are professionals, work in offices, or work at light trades expend about 4500 kcal each week on the job. Assuming a 40-hour work week, our first rough rule of thumb is that most of us burn slightly more than *100 kcal per hour* when on the job. A second rule of thumb is that those of us who are reasonably close to average weight burn about *100 kcal per mile* when walking very swiftly or jogging very slowly.[21] Runners burn about 100 to 130 kcal per mile, and walkers about 70 to 100 kcal per mile, depending on factors such as speed, temperature, humidity, terrain, and, most of all, body weight. These two rules of thumb are sobering when we consider how easy it is to wolf down 500 calories of pie or ice cream, and how tough it is to burn them off. Such a piece of pie would fuel a five-mile run or half a day's normal physical activity.

Among Harvard graduates, the protective shield of walking, stair climbing, and both light and strenuous sports activity began to take form when less than 500 kcal a week were regularly expended in these sorts of activities. Risk of death from all causes decreased steadily from slightly less than 500 kcal on up to 3500 kcal per week, where it stabilized, and where risk of death was less than half that associated with minimal activity levels.

Gains in reduced heart-attack risk were modest after about 2000 kcal per week, so Paffenbarger split his men into more and less active groups at the 2000-kcal-per-week level. Translated into activity, 2000 kcal per week works out to 20 miles of very swift walking or slow jogging. Paffenbarger found that the overall risk of death was 38 percent higher for men who regularly expended fewer than 2000 kcal per week in physical activity than for those who expended 2000 kcal or more. The greatest payoff in risk reduction came as these Harvard graduates became older. Those who were 70 to 74 years of age and very active, for example, had half the death risk of those who were the same age and very inactive. Thus it appears that physical activity becomes more critical and has a larger return the older we become.

This life-extending protective effect of exercise proves to be independent of other influences. With or without the influence of such highly significant factors as hypertension, cigarette smoking, weight extremes, gains in body weight, or early parental death, Paffenbarger's research revealed that mortality rates were lower for physically active men. For example, hypertensive men or men who smoke both have twice the death risk of those of us with normal blood pressure and those of us who do not smoke, but hypertensive men and smokers who are physically active are at significantly less risk than those who are inactive. Thus, exercise appears to ameliorate the negative effects of a risk characteristic and an antilife habit.

The Harvard study also tells us something about the consequences of exchanging a life-aversive characteristic or habit for a more healthful one. In America, the relative risks of death are greatest for hypertensive men and men who smoke. Individual men in these two groups have most to gain by stopping smoking or by achieving normal blood pressure. However, the numbers of men who suffer from hypertension are far fewer than the numbers of men who smoke and of men who are chronically inactive. So when we take a broader view, the greatest number of American men would be spared premature death if those who smoke kicked the dependency, and those who are sedentary began to exercise. *Thus, smoking and sedentarianism constitute the two largest societal health problems for men.*

When confounding influences, such as smoking and hypertension, are factored out, and we consider only the effects of physical activity, the projected Harvard figures suggest that within any age group from 35 through 70, 10 percent more of the active men (those who expend in excess of 2000 kcal per week in physical activity) will be alive. After 70 the percentage slowly tapers off.

By the age of 80, the amount of additional life attributable to exercise for the group of more active Harvard men is between one and two years. Harvard men, however, are a very special group. With the exception of suicide, where they have above-average rates, they have age-specific death rates of only about half those for white males in this country. This means that the projected one or two years of additional life are probably an underestimate of the real force of exercise for other, more typical American men.

We should also bear in mind that the additional years of life are only a small part of the story. Those of us who invite chronic illnesses by being sedentary not only live shorter lives but often spend a decade or more living with the debilitating symptoms of those illnesses. Thus the quality of life is severely impacted both physically and psychologically.

What the Harvard findings suggest is that *almost any kind of physical activity has a role in prolonging life.* Thus, some basic rules might be to stand instead of sitting, walk instead of riding, run instead of walking, and use the stairs instead of riding the escalator. We should never pass up the opportunity to burn calories. Among epidemiologists, the rule is to use it or lose it.

The Harvard study also underlines the fact that *for exercise to have an immunizing effect on heart attacks, it must be continuous.* Having been an athlete in college has no lasting effect. Only a lifestyle which incorporates regular exercise has a protective effect. This is a strong counterargument to the frequently heard contention that people who have fewer heart attacks were simply "born that way." Some were. Some weren't.

Paffenbarger, like so many of the scientists you will read about in this book, takes his findings to heart. He began to run when he was 45 and has now run the Western States 100-mile mountain race four times.

The National Centers for Disease Control reviewed 43 studies in an attempt to resolve the controversy over whether or not exercise can prevent heart disease. The agency published its findings in the July 10, 1987, issue of *Morbidity and Mortality Weekly Report,* concluding that those studies which showed no association were flawed, and that regular vigorous exercise does indeed prevent heart disease. The report pointed out that a sedentary lifestyle constitutes as strong a risk for cardiovascular disease as smoking, hypertension, or high cholesterol. Finally, since more Americans are sedentary than are at risk in other significant ways, they concluded that *a sedentary lifestyle constituted the greatest single risk to the collective hearts of America.*

Exercise and Cardiac Reserve

While nearly half of us still die from cardiovascular disease, the mortality rate, which had been steadily rising over the years, got turned around in 1967. There has been about a 2 percent decline annually since that time. Because the rate began to decrease shortly after the Surgeon General's first report on smoking, and since the decline was very broad, covering all age, sex, and racial groups, experts suggest that it has been most likely due to smoking cessation and the improved diagnosis and treatment of hypertension. The fitness boom and dietary changes might also have made a contribution.

It is clear that the protective effect of exercise results largely from its effects on our cardiovascular system. Let's examine how exercise affects this system and protects us against coronary heart disease and sudden death.

Many of our critical physiological systems adjust to what we typically demand of them. Muscles, for example, increase and decrease in size and quality in response to use and disuse. If we ask little of certain systems, we are inviting serious trouble because several adjust in the direction of diminished reserve, and these changes can result in disability or death. It turns out that our cardiovascular (CV) system is highly plastic, shrinking with disuse and expanding with regular use.

Endurance athletes have big hearts. An autopsy of seven-time Olympic-distance-runner Paavo Nurmi's heart showed it to be far greater than normal size. A similar analysis of the heart of Clarence DeMar, a lifelong marathoner who died of cancer during his 70s, showed not only unusual left ventricular development, but coronary arteries two to three times normal size.[10] The big question, of course, is: Did these men run marathons because they had been blessed with large hearts, or did they have large hearts because they ran marathons? Just how much the large hearts and coronary arteries of such endurance athletes are the result of training is not known. They could have been born that way.

Dr. David Costill, who directs the Human Performance Laboratory at Ball State University points out that when we look at the X-ray heart shadows of middle-aged men, those of trained marathoners are about half again larger than those of other men the same age. He further tells us that one reason to think that this ventricular hypertrophy is largely a function of regular aerobic exercise is that such training results in right ventricular hypertrophy in young athletes and left-side enlargement in older athletes.[10] In other words, training appears to have different effects at different ages. Established authorities, such as Dr. Peter Wood of the Stanford Center for Research in Disease Prevention, tell us that, when using noninvasive measures, it is next to impossible to distinguish the well-developed CV systems of 50-year-old men who have run all of their lives from the CV systems of those who began to run only a few years earlier.[53]

One measure of CV conditioning relates directly to our heart's efficiency as a pump. The amount of blood that is forced out of the heart with each beat is called *stroke volume*. Our genetic package will influence the dimensions of our stroke volume. A large man will ordinarily have greater stroke volume than a small woman. Costill points out that if we assume similar cardiac outputs, the differences in the sizes of heart shadows and resting pulse rates of matched normally inactive and marathon-trained men would suggest that the latter would have stroke volumes as much a 2.5 times greater than those of the normally inactive men. However, Yale University scientist Dr. Ethan Nadel reports that the increase in absolute cardiac output which actually results from prolonged physical aerobic training is more on the order of 40 percent, increasing from less than 125 to more than 150 milliliters per heartbeat.[33]

Physical activity of all kinds will affect the hearts of the participants. But the changes will reflect both the kind and the amount of physical activity. Large hearts which are the result of physical training differ from one another, and it has been demonstrated that cardiorespiratory fitness is not the same thing as physical fitness. For example, the sculpted body of a weight lifter has remarkable skeletal-muscle development, little body fat, and a heart as big as that of a marathoner. But it is a very different heart. It has been shown that the larger-than-normal left ventrical of the weight lifter is mostly muscle wall, while that of the marathoner reflects some increased muscle wall thickness but primarily reflects a larger chamber, which allows increased stroke volume.[8] Professional bicyclists have both increased muscle wall and increased stroke volume, which reflect the isometric arm exercise and the aerobic leg exercise during endurance training. *Thus, the left ventricular development reflects the kind of training engaged in by the individual.* Marathoners have large hearts but cannot lift. Weight lifters have equally large hearts but cannot run long distances. The cardiorespiratory fitness of the marathoner, which reflects large left-ventricular stroke volume, can be acquired only by aerobic endurance training.

The increased heart size, strength, and stroke volume which comes from regular aerobic exercise has some important effects, the most significant of which is a reduction in resting pulse rate. Aerobically trained hearts, which have a large stroke volume, don't have to beat so often to get the job done, and resting pulse rate is related to endurance training in a marvelously linear fashion.

A half-dozen years ago I checked the resting pulse rates of nearly 400 men and women from the Fifty-Plus Runners Association. They ranged in age from 50 to 90. The men had run an average of 32 miles a week and the women had run an average of 24 miles a week over the past eight years. An almost perfect linear relationship was found between resting pulse rate and the number of miles these men and women ran each week. At the high end was an average of 64 beats per minute (bpm) for those who ran only 1 to 10 miles per week, and at the low end was an average of 39 bpm for those few who were running 90 to 100 miles per week. The average was 54 bpm, and only 11 of the nearly 400 had pulse rates as high as what is considered average (75 beats per minute). While these figures may sound remarkable, they are are pretty standard for distance runners of all ages.

In considering this almost perfect linear relationship between weekly mileage and resting pulse rate, one might argue that the older runners who run more miles each week do so because they were born with bigger hearts which provided them with greater stroke volume and lower resting heart rates. Perhaps their ability to engage in longer runs was the result of having a big heart to begin with rather than the opposite. While there could well be some truth to this argument, longtime distance runners would in all probability smile at such a suggestion, for they have observed their resting pulse rates routinely move up and down as they modify the intensity and duration of their training. They know that their routine base mileage produces pulse rates in the 50s, that when they slack off because of injury it may move up into the 60s, and that when they boost their mileage to get ready for a marathon their resting pulse rate may drop down into the 40s.

This sort of information has application in some rather unusual settings. The Air Force, for example, is now encouraging F-16 fighter pilots to switch from aerobic exercise, such as running, to weight lifting. Running lowers heart rate and blood pressure, diminishing the pilot's ability to withstand the punishing G (gravity) forces produced by today's high-performance military jet fighters. The laid-back, distance-running fighter pilot with a low resting pulse rate and lower blood pressure is more likely to black out, destroy a multimillion dollar aircraft, and die young with very healthy arteries and a splendid heart.

But most of us don't have to worry about G forces. We need an endurance-trained heart with a big stroke volume to provide us with a reasonable heart-rate reserve—what we have in the bank to draw on in an emergency when our lives could be on the line.

To understand the concept of heart-rate reserve it is necessary to understand that our hearts can beat only so rapidly without putting us at risk. Our maximum allowable (safe) heart rate is usually considered 220 minus our age. With that in mind, let's now consider two 60-year-old men. One is a sedentary and somewhat stressed office worker with a somewhat above-average resting pulse rate of 85. His maximum allowable heart rate (220 minus 60) is 160. His heart-rate reserve (his maximum allowable heart rate minus his resting pulse rate, or 160 minus 85) is 75 beats per minute. When stressed, he has 75 beats in the bank to draw upon before he runs into his personal heart-rate limit. A second 60-year-old who engages in regular aerobic exercise also has a maximal allowable heart rate of 160, but his resting heart rate of 50 gives him a heart-rate reserve of 110 (160 minus 50). The fit 60-year-old has nearly half again more reserve than his sedentary counterpart. What this difference in heart-rate reserve reflects, of course, is stroke volume. The heart of the 60-year-old with greater cardiorespiratory fitness doesn't have to beat as often to get the job done.

Let's now put these two men in a boat in the middle of a large and isolated cold lake. Their boat sinks, and to survive they must make a long swim to shore. When our office worker's heart reaches 160 beats a minute, it may be insufficient to deal with the stress and demands of the long, cold swim. But our fit 60-year-old, by virtue of pumping far more blood with each heartbeat, might well meet the emergency with heart rates well below his heart-rate limit.

The maximum allowable heart rate for individuals who possess a high level of cardiorespiratory fitness may actually be higher than that suggested by the 220-minus-age formula which is applied to the general population of unfit individuals. Heartbeats in the bank can easily make the difference between life and death when we encounter sudden or extreme stress.

Exercise, Hypertension, and Stress

Ventricular enlargement also has some other benefits. It results in more complete emptying with each heart contraction. The same output of blood with a lower heart rate means a greater period of rest between beats, which allows the heart more time to refill with venous blood and more time for blood to flow through our coronary arteries. This effect can serve to stabilize heart rhythms. It is also one of the mechanisms which operates to reduce blood pressure in individuals who engage in regular aerobic exercise.

I frequently receive letters from older runners who report remarkable decreases in blood pressure after beginning a program of regular aerobic exercise. The letter which follows is interesting because the writer, like so many other individuals, reports that he took up aerobic training as a necessary chore in order to increase his physical endurance for another preferred sport. As is often the case, after a few months of aerobic exercise such people discover that the benefits are far more than just increased endurance. They often make it a permanent addition to their lives, or they even relegate the previously preferred sport to a secondary position. This 58-year-old man from New Jersey had run more than 21,000 miles when he wrote the following.

> I started running to stay in shape for skiing. As I got more and more into running I stopped smoking. It became painfully clear that one or the other had to go. Then about three years ago I ran into serious economic trouble and eventually lost my business. I'm convinced that the only thing that kept me from going over the deep end was running. It also brought my blood pressure down from 170/112 to 130/80, and I lost 17 pounds.

This man's reduction in blood pressure is very substantial, but the "it" which he refers to as being responsible for the changes would be more than just the running. It would also include his weight loss and his giving up cigarettes. There are a number of dietary and lifestyle changes which can function to reduce symptomatic hypertension. The sympathetic nervous system and the renal (kidney) systems involved with sodium retention play a significant role.

Treatment of hypertension with drugs is not without controversy. In a recent article[29] Dr. Norman Kaplan, chief of the Hypertension Division at the University of Texas, was quoted as saying that nearly half of the studies done on hypertension have shown that nontreated patients lived longer than those who were treated. Kaplan suggested that this may be because of the side effects of commonly used hypertensive drugs, which appear to trade one sort of cardiac risk for another. High doses of diuretics can elevate total cholesterol levels, and beta blockers can elevate plasma trigly-ceride levels as well as reduce the levels of HDL-cholesterol, a "good" kind of cholesterol I shall discuss shortly. Dr. Vincent De-Quattro, head of the Hypertension Division at the University of Southern California, was quoted in the same article as agreeing with Kaplan in suggesting that drug therapy for hypertension should be approached with considerable caution. DeQuattro's primary recommendations for hypertensive patients are to reduce weight and to begin to exercise. He recommends mild drug therapy when other interventions fail to do the job.

There aren't a large number of studies on exercise and hyper-tension, and those that have been done typically have serious shortcomings. A review of such studies reveals that exercise pro-grams result in systolic reductions of 5 to 25 mm Hg and diastolic reductions of 3 to 15 mm Hg.[46] Such changes have definite clinical implications with regard to lowering the risk of both stroke and heart attack.

It is estimated that about 80 percent of hypertensive individu-als fall within the mild hypertension range (140 to 160 systolic and 85 to 105 diastolic blood pressure), and it would seem prudent to see whether lifestyle interventions could bring the blood pressure of such individuals down into an acceptable range before introduc-ing drug therapy.

Exercise can play a fundamental role in the treatment of hyper-tension because it offers a number of benefits. The positive conse-quences of left ventrical hypertrophy have already been discussed. Weight loss is also important in the reduction of hypertension, and exercise in conjunction with dietary restraint offers the strongest intervention for weight reduction and control. While drug therapies increase blood-chemistry risk factors, exercise, we shall shortly see, can modify blood chemistry to reduce the risks of stroke and heart attack.

Psychologist Dr. Rod Dishman of the University of Georgia

has reviewed studies concerning stress and exercise.[12] He wonders whether the sorts of physiological gains outlined above, taken together with the reduced anxiety and elevated moods provided by exercise, outweigh the the potential for obsessive behavior when exercise is prescribed for classic Type A individuals: aggressive, competitive, ambitious, and impatient people who suffer from "hurry sickness." Dishman also discusses studies of non-Type A individuals which indicate that those who are metabolically fit show better stress adaptability (plasma catecholamine response) and more rapid cardiovascular recovery from psychological stress.

Exercise is now an accepted and established element in stress reduction programs. The letter from the man in New Jersey stated that exercise "kept me from going off the deep end" during a highly stressful period. My files are filled with letters from senior runners in which the central recurrent theme concerns running to preserve sanity and to enable individuals to function during stressful periods. A 51-year-old Santa Monica man who was running 60 to 70 miles each week spells it out very straightforwardly:

> For me running is a form of therapy. Running has helped me keep my sanity at a time when everything else in my life was going to pieces. It has taught me that our potentials in life are greater than we are willing to acknowledge, and also that we can endure the endless aggravations which confront us daily. I am currently under tight economic pressure with lawsuits and a business which is tottering on the edge of bankruptcy. Nevertheless I get my mileage in every day and I feel great. Running has helped me to look at life with a philosophic detachment that would have been impossible a few years ago. After a 10-mile run and a couple of beers, I feel that I can handle any hand that is dealt me.

Exercise and Our Blood Transport System

Aerobic training increases the efficiency with which we move oxygen from our lungs to the energy furnaces in our muscles and also results in improved oxygen transport from our lungs to our blood (a better ventilation-perfusion ratio). This is largely due to an increased number of red blood cells, the oxygen transport vehicles.[33] The ratio of red blood cells to whole blood in individuals who regularly engage in aerobic exercise is actually a little on the anemic side when compared to normally inactive people. However, the athletes have more blood. Our plasma reacts rather quickly to what our activity level demands. A few weeks of bed rest will temporarily reduce total blood volume to as much as 15 percent below normal. On the other hand, regular aerobic training can elevate volume an equal amount above normal. One of the ways in which we accommodate the increase in blood volume and stroke volume is through the growth of new capillaries, particularly in our muscles.

Dr. Ethan Nadel points out that this increase in absolute blood volume may be the most significant of all adaptations to physical training.[33] It results in greater heart-stroke volume, provides better delivery to muscles, and maintains high skin blood flow for cooling. It increases our ability to take in and utilize oxygen and increases our cardiac reserve. It also helps to protect against hyperthermia (heatstroke) when we are required to work hard in high temperatures.

Electrical and Plumbing Problems

Cardiovascular events such as heart attacks and strokes basically involve either electrical or plumbing problems. The carbon monoxide in cigarette smoke, for example, can create an electrical abnormality or lead to ventricular fibrillation, causing sudden death. While regular aerobic exercise normally smooths out irregular heart rhythms, it can also dangerously aggravate the cardiac arrhythmias precipitated by an inflammation of the heart muscle (myocarditis) caused by a viral infection such as influenza. Exercising hard to "sweat out" a cold which is accompanied by a fever is unwise. Heavy exercise should wait until at least 24 hours after the fever has subsided. Fortunately, we rarely suffer myocarditis with viral infections, but taking a couple days off is good insurance.

Plumbing problems can involve heart structure abnormalities or an improper coronary-artery origin on the aorta, but the most common cause of death due to plumbing problems is hardening of the arteries (atherosclerosis or arteriosclerosis).

The pipes which carry water around our house begin to plug up the day the water is first turned on. Minerals, ever so slowly, begin to accumulate on the pipe walls, gradually reducing their diameter. We can slow the process down with a water softener, but the process goes insidiously on. We don't notice the reduction in water flow for years, but the pipes suffer from chronic disease from Day 1. So it is with our arteries. The totally occluded or plugged arteries which result in strokes and heart attacks represent disease conditions which began early in our lives. Fatty streaks and fibrous plaques develop in our large arteries, and by the time many of us reach about 45, a considerable proportion of the damage has been done.

There are at least four possible ways to deal with such plumbing problems. The most common way is to deny them, to continue with a diet rich in highly saturated fats, to keep on smoking, and to remain sedentary, believing that we are one of the chosen ones who will survive a cardiovascular event should it happen to occur. With our present awareness of the etiology of heart disease, these kinds of behavior are straightfoward invitations to premature death.

There are alternatives. One is to accept the fact that mortality statistics do in fact apply to us, and to begin to pay attention to our lifestyle in order to stop the buildup of deposits in our pipes from getting any worse. We may be able to get along just fine with the blood flow we currently enjoy. There are two other possibilities to perhaps make things better. The first is to clean the deposits off the walls, and the second is to increase the diameter of our pipes so that the deposits on the walls don't matter all that much. Let's have a look at how exercise might relate to these solutions to our plumbing problems.

Cholesterol: The Good, the Bad, and the Ugly

The first intervention involves stopping or slowing down the buildup of deposits on our arterial walls. This buildup has largely to do with two essential fatty substances, triglycerides and cholesterol. Cholesterol is an essential substance which we need for building and repairing cell membranes, building sex hormones, and helping us with digestion. Triglycerides are dietary fats which our cells either use for energy or store for future utilization. Since these substances must get transported around our bodies, and since fat doesn't dissolve in water-based blood plasma, they get packaged, with protein, into very tiny particles called *lipoproteins*.

Within the framework of arterial disease, these fatty substances come in three categories; the good, the bad, and the ugly. The ugly are the low-density lipoproteins (LDL), which deliver cholesterol to our cells. High levels of LDL in our blood are consistently associated with arterial disease and heart attacks. The Bad fats are the trigylicerides. Their role in coronary heart disease is not entirely clear, but evidence suggests that low levels are preferable.

Cholesterol, which is manufactured in our livers and taken in through our diets, is packaged with triglycerides into very-low-density-lipoprotein (VLDL) carriers and circulated through our bloodstreams. After releasing triglycerides, these now cholesterol-rich particles become LDL (low-density lipoprotein). As they pass through our arteries and veins, protein receptors on the surface of the cell walls take whatever cholesterol they require. Normally, excess LDL is then returned to the liver, converted to bile acids, and excreted. But when we overindulge in foods which are rich in saturated fats and cholesterol, our systems cannot deal with the dietary excess of triglycerides and cholesterol. The vehicles (chylomicrons) which carry the excess cholesterol and triglycerides out of the intestines overwhelm the liver, and it is unable to effectively deal with the LDL overload. The excess LDL then begins to circulate through our arteries. Unless this flood of LDL is controlled, plaque begins to form on our arterial walls and can eventually result in a heart attack or stroke. Lucky for us, there are some good guys working on our side to deal with the flood of LDL which results when we overindulge in the sorts of foods which can kill us.

The good guys are the high-density lipoproteins (HDL), the smallest and most dense of the cholesterol transport vehicles. More than a decade ago it was discovered that *people with higher levels of HDL cholesterol had fewer heart attacks*. Women (from puberty through menopause), Greenland Eskimos, dogs, and rats, for example, all have higher-than-average levels of HDL and are more resistant to heart attacks. HDL appears to act as a scavenger or garbage truck which scours our arterial walls. HDL picks up excessive and potentially dangerous cholesterol and returns it, with the help of VLDL carriers, to the liver for disposal.

While total cholesterol count can be used as a predictor of heart attack risk, the ratio of HDL to total cholesterol (TC) is thought by experts such as Dr. William Castelli, director of the famous Framingham Heart Study, to be an even better predictor.[17,20] The TC/HDL-C ratio can be altered by many things. Even light smoking by adolescents makes their cholesterol ratios look like those of high-risk elderly people. Teenagers who smoke aren't likely to suffer heart attacks, but the altered cholesterol fractions will contribute to atherosclerosis. On the other hand, exercise raises the percentage of HDL and lowers the TC/HDL-C ratio (total cholesterol divided by HDL cholesterol) to a low-risk profile. People who have an average risk of heart attack have a TC/HDL-C ratio of about 5.0. The twice-average risk is close to 10.0. Half-average risk is around 3.4.[52]

Just exactly what constitutes a safe adult total cholesterol level is not clear, but it is likely to fall below 200 milligrams per deciliter (mm/dl) range. About half of the heart attacks in America occur in those of us with TC levels below 245 mg/dl, and Castelli's Framingham study reveals that 40 percent of heart attacks in that community occurred in individuals whose total cholesterol levels were within the 200 to 240 range. No one in the Framingham study with a total cholesterol count of 150 or less has ever had a heart attack.[20] Each 1 percent drop in TC count reduces heart attack risk by 2 percent.

HDL expert Dr. Peter Wood of Stanford[25,51–58] tells us that a combination of dietary change and exercise can both reduce our TC and increase our HDL. Wood, together with his colleagues Drs. John Farquhar and William Haskell, studied a group of men and women between the ages of 35 and 59 who had run at least 15 miles a week for a minimum of one year and found them to have an average TC/HDL-C ratio of 3.1, which represents extremely low risk. These runners had high average weekly mileages (the men 40 miles and the women 35 miles), but there is considerable research which suggests that less intense and prolonged exercise programs can result in substantial increments in HDL.[52]

Drs. Wood and Haskell reviewed studies concerning exercise and HDL a decade ago and concluded that the studies consistently revealed that exercise was associated with reductions of triglycerides and LDL, and with increases of HDL.[56] More recently Dr.

Robert McCunney of Boston University has reviewed such investigations and reports that significant HDL cholesterol increments have been found in longitudinal studies in which the participants' exercise has included walking, jogging, calisthenics, and weight lifting.[28] McCunney reports that modest HDL increases (10 to 12 percent) have resulted from as few as 13 to 26 weeks of walking or jogging.

However, a Stanford research group that did a careful study of 81 healthy sedentary men who were aged 30 to 55 found that those who were randomly assigned to an exercise group had to reach a threshold mileage of at least 10 miles a week and maintain this weekly mileage for a minimum of nine months before their HDL fractions began to change. Fitness improved and body fat decreased in these men before the HDL effect was significant. When the HDL levels did increase, the amount of change was substantial (8.0 mg/100 ml), about twice what other studies have reported after shorter periods of exercise. One very interesting finding was that those men who had higher HDL levels before exercise began were more easily persuaded to run more miles.[51,57]

Experts do agree to some extent as to the amount of exercise required in order to promote an HDL effect. At least their recommendations cover a reasonably small range. Drs. Wood[51] and Hartung[18] contend that we can get a significant HDL effect in untrained men with as few as 10 or 11 miles of jogging each week. Dr. Castelli[20] concurs that 10 or 11 miles may do the job, but just to be on the safe side, he runs a minimum of 15 miles per week. Dr. Terry Kavanagh[20] contends that 20 kilometers (12.4 miles) is the minimum. Taken together, these bottom-line estimates are rather similar. What these experts have to say is that about 1000 to 1500 kcal per week regularly expended in moderately intense exercise is required for a significant HDL effect that will modify heart attack risk.

Drs. Wood, Castelli, Paffenbarger, Cooper, Sheehan, Nadel, and so many others who write about and do research on exercise and cardiovascular disease take their research findings seriously. They are all fond of HDL, and they all run. Wood, now in his late 50s, has run more than 100 marathons and has logged well in excess of 100,000 miles.

I don't have an encouraging family history with regard to heart attack statistics. My father and his brothers all died of heart disease, and a younger brother has had a heart attack. What's worse is that my TC count typically falls in the 215-to-220 area, which is within the borderline risk area (200 to 239). However I have attended to my TC/HDL-C fraction by giving up cigarettes, shedding 60 pounds, following sensible dietary guidelines, and running 30 to 35 miles each week. So while my total cholesterol count always seems to hover in the borderline risk zone, my TC/HDL-C fraction is always below 3.0 by virtue of HDL counts of around 80. Such a fraction is nearly out of sight on the low risk end of things.

In addition to being affected by exercise, HDL levels are also associated with dietary changes and weight. Higher carbohydrate intake will lower HDL levels. Switching from a saturated fat diet (red meat, butter, and tropical vegetable oils such as coconut and palm) to one where polyunsaturated oils (such as safflower or corn oil) or monosaturated oils (such as olive or peanut oil) are substituted can dramatically lower total cholesterol levels. Smoking lowers HDL levels and moderate alcohol consumption raises them. People who drink moderately outlive those of us who never use alcohol, but drinking alcohol is not a recommended way to alter HDL.

Weight loss is also associated with increased HDL levels. An analysis of relevant studies has suggested that exercise-induced HDL elevation might actually result from weight loss and body-fat-percentage adjustment, since exercise without weight loss and a change in body composition results in more modest HDL elevations.[47] This might be why HDL fractions seem to respond more dramatically to exercise in people who have been sedentary (and are likely to carry around more body fat).

A very interesting study which bears on this issue was carried out at Stanford.[58] Dr. Wood and his colleagues compared two different approaches to weight loss. Middle-aged sedentary men were randomly divided into diet and exercise groups. Over the course of a year, the dieters reduced their energy intake (by eating a smaller amount of their regular foods) but did not increase their energy output through exercise. The exercisers, on the other hand, increased their energy expenditure (mainly by running) but did not decrease their energy intake. At the end of the year both groups had significantly lowered triglyceride levels and increased HDL levels. The amounts of such changes were not different for the two groups, but a control group showed no changes in triglycerides or HDL. Thus, diet and exercise appear to elevate HDL levels equally well. But there was an important difference between the two groups. While both the dieters and the exercisers lost total body weight and fat weight, the dieters also lost lean body weight (muscle mass). The exercisers showed no such loss.

Old Pipes

There is a reasonable possibility that those of us who have lived active lives will have accumulated fewer deposits on our arterial walls than our sedentary brothers and sisters. Lowered TC and elevated HDL have been shown to slow down or halt the growth of fatty deposits on our arterial walls. But what about those of us who find ourselves still alive at age 50, after a considerable amount of the damage may already have been done? Actually most of us seem to get along rather well even with a 50 percent obstruction of coronary arteries. But can a change in lifestyle and altered cholesterol levels undo any of the buildup on our arterial walls? Can we somehow reverse arterial disease?

Research to answer these questions definitively is sketchy at this juncture. It appears unlikely that altered cholesterol levels are going to impact complicated connective-tissue-fibrotic lesions in our arteries, but some of us, perhaps one out of six, have shown a shrinkage of lipid deposits in response to favorably altered cholesterol levels.[20] The good news, of course, is that a change in lifestyle can slow down or stop further arterial constriction due to fatty buildup. More good news is that physical activity intensifies fibrinolytic activity—the dissolving of potentially dangerous blood clots.[39] It is never too late to take charge, and all is not lost if we cannot somehow scrape all the old deposits off our arterial walls. There is another possible solution to the problem of old, partially occluded plumbing.

Big Pipes

If we want to increase the blood flow in our coronary arteries, another solution would be to make the pipes bigger. Even a slight increase in diameter dramatically increases blood flow. Autopsies reveal that a few old men who have died after a lifetime of marathoning appear to have very large coronary arteries. Even with heavy fatty deposits on the walls, such large pipes make a coronary infarction next to impossible. The problem, of course, is that we don't know if these men ran marathons all of their lives because they had big pipes or vice versa. To search for clues we must look at the controlled research which has been done on our primate relatives.

Dr. Dieter Kramsch and his Boston University research team studied a group of male macaque monkeys over the course of 3½ years.[23] These Boston macaques all shared the same bland diets of monkey chow and bananas. At the beginning of the experiment they were randomly split up into three groups. One group was sedentary. A second group was sedentary and in addition dined on diet supplements of artery-plugging fat and cholesterol. A third group was physically active, but during the final 24 months of the experiment also dined on the same artery-plugging supplements fed to the second group. The active macaques spent an hour jogging in a treadmill three days a week during the entire 3½ years.

When the experiment ended, autopsies revealed that the active monkeys, in spite of a fatty diet, had significantly larger heart muscles, fewer fatty deposits in their coronary arteries, and wider arteries. It appears that young monkeys who jog can be careless about their diets and still not worry about bypass surgery. Does this mean that young human beings who jog develop wider arteries? Not necessarily. Does it mean that older monkeys or older humans develop wider arteries? Again, we don't know. But that the possibilities exist would argue strongly against a sedentary lifestyle.

The Issue of Cardiac Normality

Considering the impact of exercise on our hearts, it is important to remember that hypertrophied hearts, lower blood pressure, lower pulse rates, greater blood volume, higher HDL concentrations, and greater cardiac reserve are the norm for people of all ages who regularly engage in aerobic exercise. Chronologically old men and women who are fit enjoy relatively youthful cardiovascular ages. Primitive bushmen as well as our physically fit, long-lived contemporaries in high mountain communities where cardiovascular disease is virtually unknown share these aberrant cardiovascular systems, and the same may have been the case for early *Homo sapiens sapiens*. *What is now considered aberrant might approximate normalcy for our more physically active ancestors.*

We have always possessed highly plastic cardiovascular systems which would adjust in the direction of either increased or decreased demands, but historically it has been our nature to be active. Sedentarianism is little more than a century old in America. Our integrated systems may require regular exercise for normal functioning, and a healthy cardiovascular system may very well be exercise-dependent. Our contemporary sedentary ways may not provide us with the heart-rate reserve which characterized us during all but our most recent past. The aberrant cardiovascular systems of those of us who live physically active lives cuts the odds of suffering the premature, lethal consequences of American sedentary normality.

It turns out that men and women who exercise regularly are aberrant in a number of other life-enhancing ways.

Osteoporosis

Osteoporosis (porous bones) is serious business here in America. We all lose bone mass with age, and this loss is severe enough to cause 1.3 million bone fractures annually. This problem is especially serious for postmenopausal women, who begin to lose bone mass sharply when estrogen production ceases. One in four American women over the age of 65 suffers from osteoporosis. The result can be spongy backbones which crumble and result in dowager's hump, or broken hip bones, which can result in disability and life-threatening complications as we grow older.

A number of studies now suggest that calcium supplements alone won't prevent the occurrence of osteoporosis, at least after our bones have reached peak density in adulthood. Once bone-mass loss begins, supplemental calcium, a great deal of supplemental calcium, and no calcium at all frequently have the same depressing effect: bone-mass loss has not been stopped.[15] Calcium supplements in combination with delayed-release sodium fluoride do appear to reduce the tiny fractures which collapse spinal bones as well as to restore mass to those structures, but these supplements may actually worsen the form of osteoporosis which is found in the dense hard bones of hips.[27] However, these critical weight-bearing bones respond to a combination of calcium supplements and a low dose of estrogen (0.3 milligrams daily).[45]

But bone-mass loss need not be an inevitable part of growing old. Our skeletal system also adheres to the "use it or lose it" dictum. If we don't use our bones, they become porous and brittle. If we use them they become more dense and strong. This gain-loss process takes time—maybe not so much time in gravity-free space, but for most of us here on earth, it takes quite a while. For example, bed rest for 36 weeks results in bone-mass loss equal to that lost over a normal 10-year aging span.[30] One researcher suggests that, in the case of our important weight-bearing bones, we need to be on our feet at least three hours a day just to break even.[4]

If we want the weight-bearing bones in our legs, hips, and spines to do a life-long job for us, we must use them. This particularly critical group of bone structures was shown to have much greater bone-mineral content in a group of 50- to 59-year-old male cross-country runners (with 25 years of running experience) than in a second group of previously sedentary men who had trained physically for only three months,[11] and male marathoners have been shown to have greater skeletal mass than normally sedentary men.[1]

A Stanford research team has recently taken a look at the bone density in members of the Fifty-Plus Runners Association. These 50- to 72-year-old male and female distance runners, who averaged about 25 miles per week, had about *40 percent more bone mineral* (CAT scan of the first lumbar vertebra) than normally active men and women of the same ages. We should take special note of the ages of these active men and women with the unusually dense bones, bearing in mind that many of them didn't begin to run until they were in their 50s or 60s. Perhaps osteoporosis is not just the natural consequence of aging.[26]

It has been shown that baseball players have more mineral content in their throwing arms than in their nondominant arms.[48]

Other sport-specific findings suggest that the kind of activity in which we engage is important if we are concerned about the health of our skeletal system.[50] Swimming, for example, can provide superb cardiovascular conditioning, but is a nongravity activity and does not provide the weight-bearing bone stresses offered by walking or running. Regular walking would seem to be a very important activity for postmenopausal women who wish to maintain strong hip bones.

Significant increases in bone density take time. Previously sedentary male office workers showed no increases after three months of regular running.[11] However, a recent study has focused on a group of men, aged 38 to 68, who had no previous formal running experience. These normally sedentary men decided to engage in nine months of training and to take part in the Honolulu Marathon.[50] The bone mineral content in the runners' heels was checked before and after the nine months of training. Similar measurements were made in a matched group of nonrunning men. The men who ran consistently were found to have significantly more dense bones after the nine months' training period, and the increases in density were directly related to the amount of total mileage each man had run.

Because of dietary restriction and abnormalities, young women who suffer from anorexia nervosa often have weak, porous bones, and some physicians recommend activity restriction. However, some anorexic women who exercise regularly and vigorously suffer little or no bone loss. Dr. Charles Chestnut of the University of Washington has recently sounded a cautionary warning for extremely lean women.[38] His research suggests that, while exercise per se is beneficial to bones, women who exercise enough to disrupt their menstrual periods may suffer an irreversible loss of bone mass. Chestnut reports cases where even when ammenorrhea terminated (periods resumed) after women cut back the distance they were running each week, the bones of some women didn't seem to recover fully. Ammenorrhea is most common among runners, cyclists, swimmers, and ballet dancers, and it appears to involve the interaction of nutrition, stress, and exercise. Whatever the causal contributors, exercising beyond ones individual threshold and disrupting menstrual periods appear to carry a certain amount of risk.

However, all the news is not disheartening. Several studies have now demonstrated that even mild regular exercise may delay bone loss or promote bone formation in elderly women who are most at risk for osteoporosis.[2,42,43]

What all of this suggests is that *the bone loss which afflicts us in older age is partially the result of an unnatural lifestyle rather than the natural consequence of the aging process.* Men and women who remain physically active into old age are not likely to suffer from osteoporosis. A normal diet and moderate regular exercise should keep the skeletal systems of most of us in fine shape. For those of us who may require calcium and estrogen supplements, exercise may be a viable adjunctive prescription which can reduce the amount of estrogen required. Bones need more than drugs and diet supplements to remain strong. Drugs should not be used in order to permit us to live an unhealthy and unnatural lifestyle.

Osteoporosis and Protein Intake

Countries, such as the United States and New Zealand, where people consume unusually large quantities of meat have among the world's highest rates of osteoporosis and hip fractures. Eskimos have less dense bones than Caucasians who live in the same areas, but who eat less protein.[5]

We are designed to be active carbohydrate burners, and our primary fuel is sugar, not protein. Protein can contribute to our energy, but it comes into play only in very protracted endurance kinds of activities. Carbohydrates are a clean-burning fuel which leaves behind only benign water and carbon dioxide, but the metabolism of protein leaves nitrogen and several other toxic substances which put a significant strain on our kidneys.[49] Long-term high-protein diets may cause kidney damage.[5] Breaking down protein also requires a great deal of water, leaving us dehydrated. But central to this discussion is that fact that the more protein we eat, the more calcium our kidneys excrete. Doubling our protein intake can increase calcium loss by 50 percent. If we want strong bones it is unwise to be sedentary or to eat a high-protein diet. Regular moderate exercise and a sensible diet will do the job.

Most of us don't require more than two or three ounces of protein daily, and we don't have to find it in red meat, which carries other risks.

If you have an interest in your personal protein needs, the World Health Organization's rather generous recommendations for minimal daily protein requirements are: our weight in pounds multiplied by .259 for men and .236 for women. The resulting figures are in grams (there are 28 grams in an ounce). The U.S. Department of Agriculture points out that young children (aged 1 to 3 years) need an average of about 23 grams daily. Protein needs gradually increase as we attain adulthood when the average woman requires 44 grams and the average male requires 56 grams daily.

Protein, by the way, does not simply translate into ounces of meat. A well-trimmed steak contains about 50 percent fat, and a choice T-bone may be as much as 80 percent fat. It is a wise thing to read labels. Almost everything contains protein, and there are safer places to get it than in red meat. A single quart of nonfat milk, for example, contains 36 grams of protein.

Diabetes

Dr. Walter Bortz II is a Palo Alto gerontologist who lectures and writes extensively about aging and disuse.[6,7] Bortz believes that aging takes the blame for many disorders which are actually the result of disuse, and like other scientists who do research on lifestyle consequences, Bortz practices what he preaches. He, too, is a distance runner.

Bortz points out that exercise can partially ameliorate the effects of Type I diabetes. Diabetics suffer from an insufficient supply of insulin, a substance which promotes the burning of glucose (blood sugar), and they consequently have an excess of blood glucose (hyperglycemia). Exercise burns glucose independently (without requiring insulin), allowing some diabetics to cut down on the amount of insulin they must take. The cardiovascular and weight-loss benefits which come with exercise are especially helpful to diabetics, and for them, exercise is an almost universal prescription to aid in the normalization of carbohydrate metabolism. Some individuals who have only marginally pathological conditions can be normalized with exercise alone.

Cancer

The jury which is deliberating on the relationship between exercise and cancer is still out. It may be out for some time since there is so little evidence to consider. A recent review by Michele Gauthier, an associate editor of *The Physician and Sportsmedicine*, finds that the relevant studies are few and frequently flawed.[16]

Gauthier points out that physically active people have more frequent bowel movements than sedentary people. Runners, for example, report that they never suffer from constipation, a condition which is associated with increased risk of colon cancer (probably because the intestine has more time to be in contact with carcinogenic fecal matter). Gauthier reviewed three studies which reported a higher incidence of colon cancer in people who worked on sedentary jobs, but these studies didn't report what else these people did in the way of exercise. While these findings are in the predicted direction, they do not constitute convincing proof that exercise reduces colon cancer risk.

One report has suggested that exercise might actually be an indirect cause of colon cancer.[44] The research suggested that colon cancer risk increased as serum cholesterol levels were reduced, and that high levels of HDL were positively related to that increased risk. Just when we have all been trying to change our eating habits to reduce our cholesterol, and have begun exercising to boost our HDL, along comes this unsettling bit of news. However, a more recent investigation at California's Kaiser Permanente Hospitals found no relationships of any kind between serum cholesterol levels and colon cancer.[41] Whatever future research reveals, it would seem that reduction of heart attack risk might be paramount if a choice of risks were forced upon us. Cardiovascular disease kills half of us, but colon cancer kills a considerably smaller fraction.

Dr. Steven Blair, director of epidemiology at the Institute of Aerobics in Dallas, has reported that a preliminary look at data collected on more than 250,000 armed-service veterans suggests that those who were more physically active on the job (since 1950) had lower rates of colon, brain, and kidney cancer, as well as lower rates of leukemia.[40] However, the more active veterans appeared to have higher rates of stomach cancer.

While the relationship between exercise and cancer remains ambiguous at this point, more than a half-dozen forms of cancer are clearly related to obesity. Obesity is related to higher rates of colon, prostate, breast, pancreas, ovary, endometrium, gallbladder, and kidney cancer. With regard to cancer, it may well turn out that the beneficent effects of exercise might largely result from how it impacts weight control.

Exercise and Weight Control Problems

Fat can be both a blessing and a curse. It was an ancient lean-times asset but has more recently become a Good Life liability.

In the distant past, our survival depended on fat for a number of reasons. Those reasons are related to the sources of our energy. It turns out that we have two basic sources of fuel. We burn (oxidize) sugar (the glucose in our blood and the glucose stored as glycogen in our muscles) and we burn fat. When we are at rest we burn about 90 percent fat, but as we become active we run on a blend of fuels. The changes in energy sources which take place during very moderate exercise (30 to 60 percent Vo_{2max}) follow a pattern.[3] At first, muscle glycogen is our major fuel source, but with sustained exercise, blood glucose becomes increasingly important. When our liver can no longer supply enough glucose to keep up with demand, fatty acids provide the major source of fuel. Fatty acids provide about 40 percent of our energy for the first two hours of very moderate exercise; then their contribution rapidly increases, reaching over 60 percent after four hours.

When exercise intensity is elevated to a level which can result in aerobic conditioning (65 percent Vo_{2max}) and is held stable on a treadmill, the increased fat-fuel utilization begins much earlier. For those of us who are interested in losing or controlling weight, this is good news. Dr. David Costill found that after 10 minutes of exercise at this sustained moderate intensity, fats contributed 39 percent of total energy, but that its contribution then increased in a reasonably linear fashion up to 67 percent at the end of the two-hour test.[10]

Historically, our survival depended on our capacity for two sorts of physical activities. First, we needed to be able to react intensely to emergencies. These acute "fight-or-flight" bursts of activity are fueled by sugar. Our survival also hinged on our capacity for endurance, and these long, sustained efforts were largely fueled by fat.

Besides being a vital fuel source, fat had other evolutionary advantages. It allowed for economical storage of great energy reserves which would get us through times when food was scarce. A pound of fat contains 4800 calories, and a pound of fat tissue contains 3500 calories, whereas a pound of glucose contains only 1920 calories. If we fattened up in the fall, not only would we have energy reserves on which to feed during lean times, but we were also better insulated against winter's cold. We stood a better chance of welcoming spring, shivering and skinny, but alive. Women would cease ovulating when their body fat dropped down around 10 percent, and began again when they had a better chance to sustain both themselves and a baby.

The ability to store fat became a mixed blessing in this country when our lifestyle began to diverge sharply from that for which we were designed. The relative abundance of food and the development of all sorts of food preservation techniques made life-sustaining energy available to us the year around. Television commercials constantly reminded us that there were all of those marvelous things in the kitchen, and that, with little effort, we could even send out and have something delivered, piping hot.

While our need to store fat in our bodies diminished, our capacity to do so did not. It is estimated that between 40 and 80 million Americans are seriously overweight.[22] In 1985, a National Institutes of Health (NIH) panel defined obesity as being 20 percent over the desirable weight set by life insurance tables, and many authorities now believe that the current standards (Metropolitan Life) are set too high. The NIH panel pointed out that 34 million of us are so overweight that we have put ourselves at significantly higher risk of death.[34] Those of us who are 20 to 30 percent overweight have mortality rates 40 percent higher than people of normal weight, and as our obesity further increases, so do our mortality rates. Those of us who are obese die earlier from cardiovascular disease and a host of cancers. We suffer more from hypertension, diabetes, and osteoarthritis. We are high surgical risks. Being fat also often has negative psychological consequences related to self-esteem and depression in this society where thinness is prized. And pragmatically, when we become very overweight, we frequently become nonparticipants in many of life's activities.

Eat More and Weigh Less

There are two ways to get rid of excess fat. It can be surgically reduced in a variety of ways, or it can be burned. We are going to talk about burning fat, and since more than 90 percent of our fat is burned in the furnaces of our muscles, it stands to reason that a logical place to look for answers to the problem of excess fat is in the muscles, and in increased activity levels.

Dr. Peter Wood and the Stanford group that compared the HDL fractions of distance runners to those of men and women of the same age who were chosen at random from the same community also studied the participants' dietary intake. The most striking differences between the active and the control groups were that the *active people ate more and weighed less*.[54,55]

Both male and female runners ate about 600 calories per day more (about 25 percent more) than their less active counterparts. Six hundred calories a day pretty much accounted for the caloric requirements of their average 35 to 40 miles of running per week.

The runners were also lean. This does not mean that they were all reed thin. Runners come in all shapes. What it means is that they carried low percentages of body fat. The men averaged 13 percent body fat and the women averaged 21 percent. These percentages are close to their ideal lean body weights. The randomly chosen sedentary men and women averaged 21 and 32 percent body fat. The men carried one of each five pounds of body weight as fat, and the females carried almost one of each three pounds as fat. Not healthy.

Metabolic Rates and Afterburners

What is it about distance running and distance runners that results in their being able to eat more and weigh less? Is it just because of the extra calories burned while exercising, or could it be that they are blessed with higher resting metabolic rates and are just naturally great caloric furnaces? Actually, genes appear to play a minor role in determining our resting metabolic rate, but this whole topic of metabolic rates is controversial and unsettled. For example, it's commonly thought that those of us who are overweight are cursed with lower resting metabolic rates and naturally reduced energy expenditure. But one review of many studies concludes that just the opposite is often true. One study, for example, found that overweight individuals typically have resting metabolic rates about 20 percent higher than those who are lean.[35]

However, a second reviewer reports that one expert has concluded that the primary determiner of metabolic rate appears to be the percentage of our fat-free body mass. The greater our percentage of muscle, the higher our metabolic rate. This would appear to make sense, since nearly all of our calories are burned in our muscles.[25]

Physical inactivity itself does not lower our resting metabolic rates. Quadraplegics, for example, do not have lower metabolic rates than normal individuals. However, physical activity consistently raises our metabolic rates. The lean Stanford runners we discussed burned off an extra 4000 or so calories a week while exercising.

While there is no question about metabolic rate being elevated during exercise, there is considerable debate about whether above-normal rates persist after exercise ceases. Many researchers have contended that there is such a thermogenic "afterburn" effect, which may last for hours after we cease exercising, causing us to burn calories at a higher rate. A review of more than a dozen studies points out that the most widely quoted studies which support the notion of a lasting thermogenic effect had questionable design and measurement problems. A recent study demonstrated that very intense exercise (90 percent $Vo_{2_{max}}$) to exhaustion is followed by significantly higher thermogenic activity for only about 15 minutes. Of the nine most recent and best designed studies reviewed, eight showed no prolonged thermogenic effect.[35]

Another reviewer has discussed a series of interesting studies at Laval University in Quebec.[25] The Canadians discovered that when exercise is either *prolonged* or *very strenuous*, the resting metabolic rate remains somewhat elevated for from 24 to 48 hours afterward. They also found that both nonoverweight (20 percent body fat) and moderately overweight (32 percent body fat) women who did aerobic training five hours a week over the course of 11 weeks raised their resting metabolic rate by about 8 percent. A sobering finding was that when highly conditioned distance runners refrained from exercise for only three days, their resting metabolic rates dropped almost 7 percent. If, in fact, very strenuous or prolonged exercise can effectively keep us burning calories at a higher-than-normal rate for many hours after that exercise ceases, there is an obvious Catch-22 involved. Those of us who are most overweight and would most benefit from this thermogenic afterburn effect are not capable of doing the sort of exercise which will promote it. However, everyone who exercises burns calories at higher rates while exercising, and the long-term benefits of exercise include a gradual substitution of lean body mass for fat mass and might effectively elevate our resting metabolic rate.

More and Bigger Fat Furnaces

Another factor which operates to keep active people lean is that they become more efficient fat-burners. We have seen that the longer we engage in a session of aerobic exercise, the greater is the contribution of fat to our total fuel consumption. Recall Costill's research,[10] which demonstrated that after moderate-intensity running for 10 minutes, fatty acids contribute about 40 percent of our energy. By 30 minutes they contribute about 50 percent, and by two hours their contribution is more than 65 percent. It follows that if our goal is to burn off fat, exercise should be moderate, steady, and prolonged. The longer we continue a given period of exercise, the greater the payoff. But there is more. If we exercise with regularity, we can actually restructure our muscles for another sort of payoff.

This second payoff has to do with the muscle cell powerhouses or furnaces which are responsible for oxidizing fuel. They are called *mitochondria*, and Costill points out that our muscles' reaction to continued, regular aerobic exercise is to increase both the number and the size of these furnaces. This adaptation to regular exercise enables our muscles to substitute fatty acids as an energy source for sustained endurance, and to conserve a supply of glycogen to deal with acute emergencies. These effects had obvious evolutionary advantages. Early humans, tired after a long day of physical activity, had the glycogen reserves for the acute energy demands of a fight-or-flight emergency. This sort of reserve allows today's marathoner to "have something left" for the final sprint to the finish line after running nearly 26.2 miles. For those of us interested in losing and controlling weight, this increased number of larger fat-burning furnaces is the best sort of news.

Regular aerobic exercise also reinforces the mechanisms responsible for breaking down fat cells and releasing burnable fatty acids to be used in our fat furnaces. Costill reports that the muscles of individuals who exercise regularly may contain more than three times the mitochondrial oxidative enzymes (succinic dehydrogenase) found in the muscles of untrained individuals. The overall gain is remarkable. After marathon training, for example, our calf muscles may be seven times more capable of burning fat than untrained muscles. The fat-burning capacity of our muscles is clearly a function of the volume of work they are regularly asked to perform.[10]

Besides long runs, or the aerobic equivalent, Costill's research tells us there is another way to trick our muscles into burning more fat. You will remember that free fatty acids are ordinarily released and burned at higher rates during later stages of sustained physical activity. However, if these free fatty acids are available at earlier stages, we will utilize them as fuel and conserve some of our glycogen. Exercise raises the levels of both dopamine and norepinephrine, and they, in turn, serve to release fatty acids. The trick is to find a way to raise the levels of these two catecholamines earlier. Costill's secret is coffee.[9]

His research suggests that two cups of coffee (with caffeine) taken one hour prior to exercise will increase our time to exhaustion and will nearly double the percentage of fat utilized as fuel.

As is nearly always the case, there are some trade-offs. Coffee has a mild diuretic effect, so we must be careful to drink water during very long, hot workouts. Coffee can also cause heartburn for those of us with sensitive stomachs, so our preworkout fuel should be coffee with milk, or an antacid. Coffee raises blood pressure and heart rates, and in very rare individuals it can create heartbeat irregularities. But for most of us, moderate amounts of coffee pose no significant health threat. Coffee can be a safe adjunctive tool for an exercise-based weight-control program. When I discuss two prerun cups of coffee with my students, the predictable first concern from the women runners has to do with finding bathrooms. I tell them that this problem always adds excitement, variety, and creativity to daily runs.

Exercise plus Diet for Weight Control

Attempting to lose weight through diet alone is a tough, but not impossible, proposition. Despite periodic nihilistic proclamations that diets inevitably fail and that obesity is incurable, there are studies which show that it is possible both to lose weight and to keep it off with diet alone. There is, however, an increasing number of studies which suggest that a combination of diet and exercise is superior to either diet alone or exercise alone when it comes to losing weight.

The diet-alone alternative has a number of problems. First off, the genetically programmed wisdom of our bodies reacts to food deprivation as a danger signal, and it responds in predictable ways. When food intake is suddenly reduced, our metabolic rates get dialed down as a conservation measure. This reaction is self-defeating if we are trying to lose weight.

Extreme, radical, or unbalanced dieting can cause other serious problems. Extended fasting is an extreme form of stress which can result in pronounced muscle-tissue loss, a host of nutrition-related problems, and an increase in the number of the enzymes which are responsible for laying down fat. Even when we resume normal eating, considerable time passes before these unwelcome enzymes return to normal levels. The loss of muscle mass is also self-defeating, since it is in the muscles that most of our calories are burned. Our ability to utilize fat as an energy source also diminishes. The enzymes which metabolize fat are fragile and break down, so those which burn glucose mainly take over.

Even a sensible long-term diet program can result in a loss of muscle tissue. The Stanford study which was discussed earlier showed that diet alone and exercise alone were equally effective with regard to total weight loss, but that the diet-only people lost both fat and lean body mass while the exercise-alone people lost only fat.

A first-class weight reduction program which involves both moderate diet and exercise may not reflect much change in body weight for considerable time. This is because as fat percentage is reduced, muscle tissue is being increased. Body composition and shape may change while weight remains rather constant. But slower is better in many ways. In addition to the reasons outlined above, odds are that slower weight loss is more likely to reflect permanent lifestyle change.

A University of Wisconsin study concerning metabolic rate underlines why a combination of diet plus exercise might be the best approach to weight loss.[13] It was discovered that dietary restriction reduced metabolic rate about *twice* what we would expect on the basis of the resulting weight loss. But when exercise was added, the metabolic rate was raised to levels appropriate to the prevailing body weight. Thus, the negative metabolic consequences of dieting can be countered by exercise.

The kind of exercise which is used in conjunction with diet is of real consequence, not so much for getting our weight down, but for keeping it off over the long haul. Scientists at the University of Pittsburgh conducted a long-term weight-control study of children and their parents which revealed that either formal aerobic-exercise programs or lifestyle exercise (beginning to routinely walk to school, work, shopping, and so on) can reduce weight equally well when used in conjunction with a light diet. However, the researchers found that when they checked back a year or two after the programs ended, *participants who had adopted lifestyle exercise habits were more likely to have maintained their weight loss* than those who had engaged in formal aerobic programs. Thus, it appears that a permanent change in basic lifestyle (beginning to eat a little less and incorporating routine exercise into our daily life) may hold the greatest hope for those of us who wish to weigh less.[14]

Some Final Thoughts

If we begin to exercise regularly in order to ease our troubled minds, we stand to gain in many other ways. Regular physical activity can add years to our lives and cut the risks of heart attacks. It can somewhat ameliorate the negative consequences of our other antilife habits (smoking) or characteristics (hypertension), and can add to the quality of our entire lives. Most of us don't have to live with severely compromised cardiovascular systems, weak bones, weak muscles, and excess fat. Exercise can change our moods, our bodies, and our lives. Regular physical activity was obviously an assumed factor in our genetic formula. We just don't work right without it. Being sedentary is not being human.

Chapter 11
The Risks

Exercise and Sudden Death

If we awake each morning and vow to live that day as though it is our last, one day we will be proven right. The trick is to stay alive and to live fully as many days as possible. Within this formula, exercise assumes a curious Catch-22 quality. On the one hand, it can extend our years—largely through its protective effect with regard to reducing heart attack risk. But on the other hand, we are more likely to suffer a heart attack while we are exercising (or shortly thereafter) than at those times when we are sedentary.[9,18,22] So how do we resolve this Catch-22 dilemma? There is now considerable research which provides the sort of answers which we need to make sensible decisions concerning the role of exercise in our personal lives. Let's begin with an examination of how the amount of regular exercise bears on death from sudden heart attacks.

Engaging in strenuous physical activities such as jogging, swimming, singles tennis, or chopping wood has a great deal to do with fixing the odds of a fatal cardiac arrest. A University of Washington research team headed by Dr. David Siscovick found that men who spent 2 hours and 20 minutes or more per week at these activities were 5 more times likely to suffer cardiac arrest while exercising strenuously than at other times.[24] Sounds bad. But consider the odds of those who exercised less. Those who exercised strenuously less than the most active group, but at least 20 minutes a week, were 13 times more likely to suffer sudden death while exercising. For those who exercised strenuously less than 20 minutes a week, the odds of exercise-induced sudden death were a very frightening 56 times higher.

It's clear that the benefits of exercise far outweigh the risks. If we want to avoid sudden death while exercising, the best bet is to exercise regularly. And the fact that we are more likely to suffer sudden death while exercising does not imply that the cause of death was exercise. The opposite is more likely to be the true: we are more likely to suffer exercise-induced sudden death because we don't exercise. So, if you have been allotted only three more hours until you die, and you want to live until the very last second, head for the couch. On the other hand if you have an indeterminate period of life ahead and you have an investment in being around for a while, you and the couch should become strangers.

Sudden death (death which occurs within six hours of the onset of symptoms) accounts for about one-fourth of all deaths in America each year, and 40 percent of them are the result of cardiac arrest.[5] We can take our last breath while sleeping, golfing, making love, or watching television. Just by chance alone, some of us will have a fatal seizure while running. Dr. Jeffrey Koplan of the Atlanta Centers for Disease Control has consulted the data available and worked out the probabilities.[14] If we assume that 4 million lean, nonsmoking men run 20 minutes three times a week, 4 would suffer sudden death each year just by chance alone. If we add on the two hours which follow each run, another 30 deaths would be expected. But if we assume that the runners are average white male Americans (as against lean nonsmokers) the numbers grow to 15 (while running) and another 104 (after running). Thus, chance alone accounts for from 4 to 104 sudden deaths per year for male runners. However, Koplan points out that average white male Americans will suffer such fatal seizures three to four times more frequently than lean, nonsmoking men.

Koplan's figures are especially interesting in that it appears that the two hours following strenuous exercise are more dangerous than the exercise period itself. A primary reason for these postexercise sudden deaths is that many of us do not warm down after we finish an acute bout of exercise. We simply stop, and this can be fatal. It is important to slow down or reduce the intensity of our activity over the course of a few minutes while our heart rates and blood pressures move back down to more normal levels.

When we exercise strenuously, the blood vessels which supply our muscles (including our heart muscle) dilate. If we suddenly stop exercising, our muscles cease contracting and our blood pressure plummets. Blood pools in our extremities, especially our legs, and oxygen is less available to our muscles. We feel lightheaded and can even black out. Our body responds to this crisis by suddenly boosting our dopamine and norepinephrine levels in order to restore blood pressure. The response of heightened pulse and narrowed arteries can be fatal if our coronary arteries are already dangerously compromised by plaque buildup or if we set off a heartbeat arrhythmia. The rule is never to cease exercise abruptly. We should always warm down by reducing exercise intensity until our cardiovascular system achieves a reasonably normal state. Walking for a few minutes after a hard run will do the job. So will a leisurely lap or two in the pool, or an easy final mile after a hard bike ride.

Apart from Koplan's projections of exercise-induced sudden deaths accounted for just by chance, what actually happens out there in the real world? How many people die while exercising, and just exactly who are they? Cardiac and exercise expert, Dr. Ken Cooper tells us that sudden death while exercising does not occur anywhere near as often as we might think. He discusses a review of international studies of exercise-related sudden death that reports that of 2606 sudden deaths in Finland only 22 (less than 1 percent) were associated with sports—about one-third the number which occurred in sauna baths.[5]

Some very interesting data on exercise-induced sudden death come from the state of Rhode Island.[22] During the 88-month period beginning in January of 1975, there were 81 sudden deaths which occurred during or just following recreational exercise in that state. With the exception of a single black man and one woman, the victims were all white males. Most of the men (19) died on golf courses, followed by joggers (16). Swimming (9) and bowling (6) were next in line. Most deaths occurred among 50- to 59-year-olds (30), followed by 40- to 49-year-olds (23). The deaths involved a total of 10 different sorts of cardiac and vascular disorders, but 71 of them (88 percent) were caused by atherosclerotic coronary artery disease (ACHD), a narrowing and final closing of the arteries which supply our heart muscles with blood.

Several recent investigations confirm the findings that existing ACHD is the primary culprit in sudden deaths which are related to exercise. Dr. Larry Gibbons and his associates at the Institute for Aerobic Research in Dallas kept records on exercise and cardiac events for almost 3000 adults over five years.[12] They, too, concluded that exercise per se does not cause sudden death in people with healthy hearts. Exercise places additional stress on already compromised and susceptible hearts. They also point out that besides ACHD, factors such as smoking, competition, and irregular exercise may also increase risk. Other studies have revealed that 70 percent of those who suffered sudden death while exercising were heavy smokers.[9,18]

These sorts of findings suggest two things. The first and most important is that *exercise-induced sudden death is rare*. In Rhode Island, depending on age and sex, there were between 0.05 and 4.46 such deaths among 100,000 persons each year. A single woman and only six men under the age of 30 suffered sudden death during the 88 months of that study. Second, *the cause of exercise-induced sudden death is almost always existing and advanced atherosclerotic coronary artery disease*. Exercise pulls the trigger, but the bullet is ACHD.

It follows that the older we get, the more imperative it is that we have a cardiac examination before we begin an exercise program. Exercise doesn't have to be all that strenuous to constitute risk. In Rhode Island the most exercise-induced sudden deaths struck golfers who averaged 59 years of age, and the fourth place was occupied by bowlers who averaged 57 years of age. It doesn't take much to pull the trigger if ACHD is in an advanced stage. If our coronary arteries are seriously compromised, an exercise program should be supervised.

Besides age, there are some other high-risk markers which should prompt us to have a cardiac exam prior to beginning serious exercise. Those of us with a family history of ACHD should consider a cardiac exam prior to an exercise program as early as the age of 30. Those of us who smoke, are obese, suffer from hypertension, have diabetes, have high plasma-cholesterol levels, or have survived a coronary infarction should consult with a specialist and perhaps exercise only with supervision. Even if it means traveling to another city, it is wise to consult with someone who specializes in the diagnosis, treatment, and exercise supervision of people who have the same high-risk conditions as our own. Most large cities, for example, have supervised exercise programs for those of us who have survived heart attacks, are dangerously obese, or have hypertension. We shouldn't consult just any physician about exercise. In these litigious days, conservative advice is the rule, and most general practitioners simply cannot keep up to date on all aspects of medicine. Other things being equal, seek out an appropriate specialist. Almost all of us can exercise safely, but not all of us can do so without supervision.

While ACHD is the primary killer in America and the primary cause of exercise-induced sudden death, its diagnosis is not an easy task. The only definitive way we can assess ACHD is with a coronary angiogram. Most of us are unwilling to undergo this sort of procedure, and it quite simply isn't necessary. Treadmill stress tests are not always accurate indicators (and they tend to be most inaccurate when there is the least apparent likelihood of ACHD), but they are of real value. A treadmill stress test is useful to screen for other sorts of cardiac problems, such as myocardial ischemia, hypertrophic cardiomyopathy, or ventricular rhythm disturbances. Most experts agree that a treadmill stress test should be a prerequisite to beginning a strenuous exercise program.

But when push comes to shove, the best judge of whether or not we suffer from dangerously narrow coronary arteries is ourselves. The symptoms are clear. The problem is whether or not we can face the symptoms and what they imply. Many of us are reluctant even to listen to experts. It is highly probable that the few well-conditioned runners who die from ACHD ignored clear warning signs. Autopsies reveal that experienced distance runners who died from sudden death frequently showed signs of an earlier nonfatal heart attack. Perhaps it was "silent" or not actually felt. Perhaps not. The well-known running writer Jim Fixx is a classic case. His father suffered his first heart attack at age 35 and died from a fatal heart attack at age 43. Jim had reported ominous symptoms (a tightness in his chest) for several weeks and was "planning on having it checked out" when he died on a roadside. His autopsy revealed severe coronary disease and evidence of a previous recent heart attack. Reports from New Zealand, South Africa, and here in America concur that many such sudden deaths, perhaps more than half, occur in men who were aware of the symptoms but were unwilling or unable to act on them. It is not an easy thing to look into the eye of the tiger.

Nevertheless, it won't hurt to spell out the symptoms which may portend a heart attack. New Jersey cardiologist and well-known running philosopher Dr. George Sheehan[23] lists them as chest pressure, pain, or tightness under the breastbone on up to the jugular notch. The symptoms usually go away promptly when we rest, get worse when we lie down, and feel less severe if we sit up. Such pain can occur a few minutes into a run and then disappear. Other symptoms of concern are unfamiliar fatigue or exhaustion, or a significant increase in morning pulse rate. Had Jim Fixx visited a heart specialist when he became symptomatic, he would likely have had bypass surgery and would still be alive and running.

Thus, longtime and well-conditioned distance runners invite sudden death by using bad judgment, most commonly by denying ACHD symptoms, but sometimes by racing and passing up water stops on days when both temperature and humidity are dangerously high. Runners also flirt with disaster when, after a long layoff due to illness or injury, they attempt too much too soon. Cardiac events happen to some of us then. Then there are those occasional euphoric days when we are incredibly high, totally stoked on norepinephrine, dopamine, serotonin, endorphins, perfect health, and seemingly unlimited speed and power. At those rare moments when we are cognitively impaired and sometimes feel omnipotent, we might foolishly challenge trucks and cars for who has the right of way. Silly us. Dead us. Cars and trucks always have the right of way. It is wise always to run against the traffic and to assume that drivers don't always see us. Sedentary people sometimes behave as though their bodies exist only as containers in which to transport their brains around. Endurance athletes, on the other hand, sometimes behave as though they have no brains whatsoever.

Nonetheless, the big picture is a very positive one indeed. The benefits of exercise far outweigh its risks with regard to ACHD and sudden death. Such deaths are both rare and preventable provided we use good judgment. While exercise can trigger death from coronary disease, its overwhelming effect is a protective and beneficent one. *The more we exercise, the less our chance of suffering exercise-related sudden death.*

Overuse and Osteoarthritis

To hear some experts talk, one would think that walking and running are unnatural acts. We are cautioned that we have only so many steps allotted in our lifetimes before our knee and hip joints disintegrate and turn into noisy, grinding gravel pits. Running, with those endlessly repetitive gravity forces, is particularly unnatural. When faced with the sudden appearance of a saber-toothed tiger, our ancestors never stopped to debate whether they should run and risk future degenerative lower-extremity joint dysfunction. Our ancestors did considerable running, and even more walking.

Perhaps some of us have only so many steps allotted. But there are also those of us who have run in excess of 100,000 miles, and have no joint problems whatsoever. The truth of the matter is that we simply don't know whether regular distance-running ruins our knees and hips. However, two recent cross-sectional studies make it abundantly clear that distance running need not be associated with premature degenerative joint disease (osteoarthritis) in our lower extremities.

One investigation compared a group of 60-year-old Florida men who had run an average of 17,500 miles over the past 12 years with a matched group of nonrunners.[19] There were *no differences* between the two groups with regard to degenerative joint disease from hips to toes.

At Stanford University, nearly 500 men and women between the ages of 50 and 72, who had run an average of more than 15,000 miles (27 miles a week for 11 years), were studied. These runners were compared to a similar group of matched nonrunners.[15] The groups showed *no differences* in jointspace narrowing, crepitation, joint stability, or symptomatic osteoarthritis. While the joint-space differences between the two groups were not statistically significant, the trend was in the direction of the runners having *more* joint space rather than less. The runners also had less physical disability, maintained a higher functional capacity, had fewer major medical problems, visited physicians less (even though a third of their visits were for running-related injuries), and were absent from work less than half as frequently as the non-runners.

The Stanford runners and their matched controls will be assessed a second time after five years have passed, and perhaps some clearer answers will be forthcoming. But even then, if the runners show no further joint degeneration, critics can still argue that the research proves nothing, that these old runners were a special group to begin with, people blessed with extremely fine knee joints which resisted overuse injuries. A more definitive experiment cannot be carried out. We cannot arbitrarily assign people to a group where high-mileage running on a daily basis is either demanded or prohibited. As scientists, we are forced to rely on periodic assessments of the joints of people who have chosen to run and continue to do so. These two studies[15,19] do, however, make it clear that high-mileage regular running does not cause osteoarthritis in all individuals.

In the end it will almost certainly come down to the fact that, for some of us, distance running is impossible because of genetically predisposed structural problems or a variety of pathological conditions. But others of us can run all of our lives and accumulate enormous mileage, without ill effects. Thus it is as foolish to say that running is safe for everyone as it is to say that it is safe for no one.

There are some ways to minimize lower-joint problems for those of us who choose to run. The most obvious one is to lose weight and cut down on the gravity forces. Another is to run on forgiving surfaces. Grass and natural dirt trails are the best. Dirt trails are safer since we can see the sorts of surface problems which grass can conceal. A hidden gopher hole can end running forever. We can therefore run in a more relaxed fashion and more safely on dirt than on grass. Cement should be outlawed for people who walk and run, but today's high-tech running shoes make it possible for most of us to run reasonably high mileage (perhaps 50 miles a week) on asphalt without serious mechanical problems.

Running is such an inexpensive sport that we need never risk injury by using poor-quality shoes. We should buy good ones and replace them when the cushioning begins to fade—usually long before they wear out. Shoes can still look great after 500 miles, but for some of us who are heavy or injury-prone, it may be time to throw them out and buy new, safe cushions. Some runners have closets filled with heaps of "perfectly good" shoes which they know better than to run in again, but which they cannot bear to part with.

Besides paying attention to the sort of surfaces on which we run, and being careful about the shoes we wear, there is one other very important factor which relates to minimizing joint injuries. While our joints seem to be able to tolerate endless uphill running, the downhill runs can be very dangerous. If we run downhill too fast or too frequently, we are asking for knee trouble. Usually there is plenty of warning. Our knees will tell us to back off on the downhills for a few days or more.

If we find that walking and running aggravate joints which may be susceptible to osteoarthritis, there are non-gravity sports such as swimming, bicycling, and rowing which might work out as acceptable forms of aerobic exercise. But no matter what the sport, those of us who exercise must always live with injuries. There are tennis elbows and runner's knees. A very large percentage of the injuries which endurance athletes suffer are self-incurred, the result of overuse, and could be avoided with improved judgment. Most such injuries will also heal very nicely without treatment if we stop our usual form of exercise long enough for the healing process to take place.

Whether we develop coronary artery restriction or a less lethal problem such as runner's knee, our bodies almost without exception signal us that something is wrong. Pain means *stop*. If we pay attention to such signals, damage can frequently be minimized, and healing time can be lessened. However, most of us tend to ignore such signals. We figure we will "run through" the injury. Sometimes we can, especially if the pain goes away and stays away after we warm up. But more commonly "running through" means significantly reducing the intensity, duration, and frequency of our training.

Some injuries demand that we stop altogether, and if we attempt to run through these sorts of injuries, they can become very serious—in some cases ending our running forever. When we run in pain, we always compensate in one way or another and frequently create new injuries in addition to the original one. Thus a foot problem can turn into a very serious foot problem plus a knee problem or even a hip problem. Experience is a tough teacher, and we learn the very important lessons in life only by making mistakes. If we are lucky we won't do any permanent damage the first time around.

Exercise Abuse and Dependency

Because of its many beneficent side effects, regular exercise has sometimes been labeled as a "positive addiction."[13] But others have written that regular exercise can turn into a destructive negative addiction. Dr. William Morgan has chronicled eight cases of negative running addiction, pointing out that this sort of addiction can result in irreparable physical injuries, damaged interpersonal relationships, lost jobs, and even death.[16] Extreme dependency is destructive and pathological no matter how you slice it. Being out of control and having no choices are both physically and socially devastating whether we are obsessed about exercise, being ultrathin, or our next hit of cocaine.

Both scientific journals and popular literature provide us with clinical reports which outline cases of so-called running addiction. The picture is a familiar and consistent one. Interpersonal relationships at home, at work, and socially begin to suffer when running takes top priority over everything else in life. So-called running addicts who are involuntarily forced to abstain from running go through withdrawal. They become irritable, anxious, and depressed. They also typically become restless and fatigued, suffer from insomnia, and have decreased appetites. The hard-core exercise addict will risk permanent physical disability by continuing to exercise contrary to medical advice, and when exercise places family, friendships, and the job in jeopardy. These symptoms sound similar to those we see in other forms of dependency. They don't sound positive at all.

If we turn to the American Psychiatric Association's *Diagnostic and Statistical Manual* (DSM-III), we discover that exercise addiction is not listed. In fact, *addiction* itself is a term which is no longer utilized. But a look at the chapter on "Substance Abuse Disorders" is instructive.

The DSM-III discriminates between substance abuse and substance dependency. Substance abuse involves a *pattern of pathological use* including "inability to cut down or stop use . . . continuation of substance use despite a serious physical disorder that the individual knows is exacerbated by use . . . daily use of the substance for adequate functioning." Abuse also includes *impairment in social and occupational functioning* caused by a pattern of pathological use: "Social relations can be disturbed by the individual's failure to meet important obligations to friends and family . . . occupational functioning can deteriorate if the individual misses work or school . . . the individual's life can become totally dominated by use." The final abuse criterion centers on *duration*: the pattern of behavior which interferes with social and occupational functioning must have lasted at least a month.

According to the DSM-III, substance dependence involves evidence of either *tolerance* or *withdrawal*: "Tolerance means that markedly increased amounts of the substance are required to achieve the desired effect or there is a markedly diminished effect with regular use of the same dose. In withdrawal, a substance-specific syndrome follows cessation of or reduction in intake of the substance that was previously regularly used by the individual to induce a physiological state of intoxication." The term *substance-specific syndrome* refers to the predictable pattern of behaviors which occur when a particular substance is withheld.

While exercise does not involve the use of substances, the clinical picture of so-called running addicts presented by Morgan and others fits very nicely into the framework of the DSM-III description of abuse and dependency. Certainly, a few runners abuse and are pathologically dependent upon running. But the great mass of men and women who run do not suffer from this pathological pattern of symptoms. Let's take a look at the possibility that even persistent and rather high-mileage running might involve a healthy commitment or even a healthy dependency.

Commitment and Dependency

Certainly many forms of exercise have the potential for abuse and dependency, and the focus on runners in this discussion simply reflects the availability of relevant data.

The parameters of exercise dependency have not been established. Just exactly where healthy commitment ends and abuse and unhealthy dependency begin is rather murky territory. It doesn't seem to come down to something as simple as weekly mileage or frequency of racing.[2,25] But even though the territory is ill defined, exercise-adherence expert Dr. Rod Dishman points out in a review of the literature that evidence from many areas of inquiry suggests that a state of exercise dependence does exist.[7]

One of the problems with doing research on the effects of exercise abstinence is that it's next to impossible to recruit subjects. People who exercise five or six days a week are generally unwilling to stop for the sake of scientific inquiry. There would seem to be a message in that. After two unsuccessful attempts to recruit such men and women to engage in research which involved a one-month withdrawal from exercise, one investigator was forced to settle for college students who exercised "only" three or four days a week.[1] They agreed voluntarily to stop exercising for an entire month. Nocturnal EEG (brain-wave) records revealed that these people suffered sleep disturbances after they stopped regular exercise. Deep slow-wave sleep decreased while REM sleep (during which rapid eye movement signals dream activity) increased.

Another study reveals that men and women between the ages of 21 and 54 who had run five days a week for at least a year reacted strongly to even a *single day* of running deprivation. They became depressed (as measured by psychological tests) and anxious (as measured physiologically).[25] Who knows what would happen if seven-day-a-week runners were *forced* to stop for a month?

Biochemical Issues

Dr. Wesley Sime's work with a single deeply depressed man (discussed in Chapter 6) dramatically demonstrated that changes in depressed mood paralleled exercise and nonexercise on random days, a finding which suggested that individuals react acutely to exercise deprivation with increases in measured depression. A second study which involved competitive and recreational runners showed that they were significantly more depressed during only two days of running deprivation, but that their depression scores promptly decreased after a run on the ensuing day. While these studies do not prove that a biochemical dependency state exists, Sime argues that the best explanation for the observed dramatic, acute mood-elevating reactions to exercise might best be explained by increased aminergic (serotonin, dopamine, norepinephrine) turnover in our brains.

The Issue of Cause and Effect

Biochemically based or not, there seems to be sufficient evidence to conclude that exercise dependency is a fact of life. But as in the case of most other forms of dependency, only a small proportion of habitual exercisers engage in exercise abuse and become dangerously dependent. Exercise is not inherently abusive. Even what some sedentary people might consider excessive exercise may not be abusive.

For those of us who need relief from the personal demons which dwell within us and spoil our relationships with others, there are any number of unhealthy ways to cope, things we may get involved with or obsess about in order to distract ourselves. Alcohol is a popular choice, drugs another. As youths we often shut the rest of our lives out by focusing totally on our studies, and as adults we sometimes survive by becoming workaholics, by gambling, or by compulsive sexualizing. Now add exercising.

Yet, most of us have used alcohol without becoming dependent. The same is true of those of us who have gambled or engaged in other potentially addictive behaviors. Most of us seem to be able to toil at our jobs within reasonably normal parameters without becoming workaholics. For that matter, most of us can see a psychotherapist without becoming hopelessly dependent. But a predictable small percentage of us abuse or become dependent on one or another of these things. The same is true of exercise. Most of us can safely exercise without becoming exercise junkies, but a small percentage of us will engage in exercise abuse and become destructively dependent.

When we hear that alcohol, drugs, the job, or running has ruined someone's family life, marriage, health, or career, it is important to pause and consider what is cause and what is effect, or what is the problem and what are the resulting symptoms. Millions of us drink, work, and exercise without having our lives crumble. Becoming abusively dependent on these things is usually the *effect*, or *symptom*, of some underlying personal distress. The cause is almost always underlying personal, family, work, or social problems. These are the factors which can turn use to abuse, and freedom of choice to dependency.

Dependency: Positive or Negative

Just as exercise can trigger sudden death in those of us with advanced coronary heart disease, so, too, can exercise be a destructive and potentially lethal vehicle for those of us with existing mental or adjustment disorders. Fortunately those who utilize exercise to self-destruct are few, and the odds are they would have chosen another obsession had exercise not been available and somehow right for them.

The vast majority of us who engage in regular endurance activities are not hopelessly or destructively dependent. I suspect that the symptoms of dependence may be stronger during the first year or two of regular training. It is then that we seem more likely to exhibit pronounced withdrawal symptoms when illness or injury rules out daily exercise. Most of us learn, after one or more serious injuries, that in time we will heal, and subsequent interruptions in training are likely to be taken more in stride. The millions us who exercise with regularity year after year would be better described as committed than as abusive or pathologically dependent, and the state of exercise dependence must be viewed largely as a positive force or process.

Dishman[7] views such dependence as an intrinsic and integrative motivational process which keeps us going and helps get us past the common compliance barriers which intimidate less active people. Whatever the combination of acute and chronic biochemical, cognitive, and mood factors which motivate and reinforce the state of exercise dependency, for some of us this process is a precious one. It's what keeps us going, until regular exercise becomes fixed as a permanent and positive component in our lifestyle, a component which bestows a multitude of both mental and physical health benefits.

Predisposition to Dependency

Exercise appears to have a number of reinforcing properties which affect all of us with variable effects, depending on our biological makeup, our personalities, and the amount and kind of stress in our lives. Exercise serves to center us and to distract us from life's stresses. It reduces our hostility and energizes us. Beta endorphin serves to ease our aches and pains and appears to produce euphoria in some of us. It also seems very probable that higher rates of norepinephrine and serotonin turnover occur in our brains during and following exercise, and that their antidepressant effects may be reinforcing. The tranquilizing effect of exercise is well-established, and also serves as a significant reinforcer.

It seems probable that some of us would be more susceptible to this dependency-producing process. Personality factors such as a lack of capacity to delay gratification, a need for change, and boredom susceptibility all play a role. So do strongly motivating environmental stress factors. There may also be biochemical predisposers. Let's consider three lines of biochemical research which bear on this issue.

First, there is evidence which suggests that low brain serotonergic turnover is specifically involved in obsessive-compulsive disorders. Drugs which act exclusively on serotoninergic transmission and even the common dietary amine L-tryptophan (which is the precurser forserotonin) have been shown to reduce obsessive-compulsive symptoms.[21] These discoveries are of interest to us since regular exercise may have compulsive components and may also have obsessive components, when committed exercise evolves into abusive dependency. Serotonin could play a role in exercise predisposition.

Second, a review of research concerned with biogenic amines and depression argues strongly that there are two subtypes of clinical depression which are associated with either low serotonin or low norepinephrine turnover in our brains.[11]

Finally, a large number of studies suggest that exercise significantly increases the turnover of both serotonin and norepinephrine in our brains and reduces symptomatic depression very effectively. Norepinephrine could also play a role in exercise predisposition.

While all of this research is necessarily indirect, it is growing in size and is quite consistent. On the basis of these related areas of animal and human research, I am going to suggest a possible bio-chemical explanation for predisposition to exercise dependency. This "serotonin hypothesis" incorporates the notion that regular exercise may have compulsive dimensions.

Could it be that one subgroup of us who exercise regularly could be more susceptible or sensitive to exercise's inherent motivating and reinforcing processes by virtue of having lower-than-average brain serotonergic turnover? And could it also be that others of us who become pathologically compulsive and destructively dependent on exercise suffer unusually low brain serotonergic turnover, perhaps even paired with low brain norepinephrine turnover sufficient to seriously depress us?

It may be that those of us who seem to move so effortlessly into regular exercise do so because we have a mild biochemical predisposition to compulsive behavior. Lower than normal serotoninergic turnover could also result in mild depression, agitation, and poor sleep. Perhaps some of us medicate ourselves with daily runs, channeling our moderate compulsive tendencies in a healthy direction, increasing our sertoninergic turnover, reducing our mild agitation and depression, and helping ourselves to sleep.

Others of us who suffer very severe serotonergic insufficiency may be predisposed to become pathological, ascetic running addicts who are acting out a true obsessive-compulsive disorder. If such serotonergic insufficiency is paired with significant adrenergic (norepinephrine) insufficiency these runners might also be self-medicating a biochemical depression. It would be most interesting to see whether fluvoxamine (which potently blocks serotonin reuptake without affecting norepinephrine) or clomipramine (which blocks serotonin reuptake and has a primary metabolite which blocks norepinephrine reuptake) would effectively impact the behavior of pathologically dependent runners. Whatever future research reveals, it seems probable that there could be bio-chemical as well as psychological predisposers for regular exercise.

Exercise and Psychopathology

If habitual exercisers sometimes suffer from obsessive-compulsive mental disorder, is the incidence of other forms of psychopathology higher among these men and women?

A few years ago an article in the *New England Journal of Medicine* received considerable press because it suggested that there were some clinical parallels between male "obligatory" runners and anorectics.[27] The researchers pointed out that members of both groups appeared to have a common family background, came from similar socioeconomic classes, were preoccupied with diet and the maintenance of an extraordinarily lean body mass, denied disabilities, inhibited their anger, shared high personal expectations, were depressed, were ascetic, and engaged in perfectionism to compensate for other psychological problems.

Southern California pathologist and distance runner Dr. Tom Bassler has done postmortem examinations on nearly three dozen "ascetic" male runners who died mysteriously.[17] He estimates that there may be as many as six such deaths each year in America. These unusual, consumed men put in extremely high mileage, were almost totally devoid of body fat, and engaged in radical and extreme dieting. He blames such deaths on cardiac arrest precipitated by nutritional arrhythmias. Bassler suggests that pathological runners of this sort are very rare.

While there appear to be some similarities between extreme obligatory, ascetic male runners and anorectics, there also appear to be some differences. Low-mileage runners who ran 30 miles or less per week tended to estimate their waist widths rather accurately, but those who ran more than 40 miles per week tended to overestimate their waist width, in the manner of anorectics.[26] However, the dietary behaviors and testosterone profiles of such runners were dissimilar to those of male anorectics.[4] Obligatory runners also have above-average cardiovascular fitness, while anorectics have $Vo_{2_{MAX}}$ scores well below average.

The dietary behavior of ectomorphic (thin) male collegiate distance runners, swimmers, and wrestlers reveals nothing unusual,[8,20] but eating problems are far above the expected frequencies for female ballet dancers and gymnasts.[6]

With regard to psychopathology, a cross-sectional study ("Running and Anorexia Revisited") has shown important differences between obligatory runners and anorectics on the Minnesota Multiphasic Personality Inventory (MMPI).[3] The MMPI is perhaps the most commonly used and widely accepted objective measure of psychopathology. Obligatory runners, as a group, scored within the normal range on the MMPI, and none showed more than two elevated scores. However, 50 percent of the anorexics had elevated scores on three or more scales, with depression and psychopathic deviation showing the greatest elevations. Apparently not all obligatory runners are clinically the same as anorectics.

Several researchers have reported psychotic, neurotic, and borderline personality disorders among selected habitual exercisers. Some runners have been diagnosed as neurotically obsessed or masochistic-narcissistic. It has also been suggested that some use exercise as a defense against internal and external conflicts, and that overidentification with exercise may represent an attempt to establish self-identity.[7] We could, of course, find similar extreme cases if we examined a cross section of the people who engage in almost any activity or occupation. All groups contain some of us who are periodically or even permanently troubled. It's a little difficult to assume that our close friends who exercise regularly are all silently ticking psychopathological time bombs.

Be reassured that recent cross-sectional studies show that the incidence of psychopathology among committed and possibly even dependent runners is no different from that found among people in general. On a broader scale, athletes from all sports tend to score within the normal range on personality tests. While they tend to be a bit more extraverted than most of us, they also tend to score a little above average with regard to emotional stability.

So, like all other substances and activities on which we may choose to focus our obsessions and hang our pathology, the exercise hook is ready and waiting. It is important, however, to distinguish between getting hooked and hooking ourselves. Most of us don't need to hook ourselves addictively to exercise or to anything else. Most of us won't.

While exercise is magnificently beneficent, it is not without risks. If we refuse to have a proper physical examination prior to beginning a strenuous exercise regimen, or if we deny the physical symptoms of impending cardiac disaster, we can use exercise to pull the trigger for sudden death. And if, when personal psychological distress is great, we turn our backs on professional help and become pathologically abusive of and dependent upon exercise, we may incur serious physical injury and jeopardize our social, family, and vocational lives.

Fortunately only a small percentage of us suffer those sorts of disastrous consequences. Exercise is not inherently dangerous or abusive. There were no shiny red sneakers hanging from the limbs of that tree in the Garden of Eden. Sneakers just go between our feet and the ground.

Chapter 12

Self-Prescription

Whether it's the daily accumulation of little things or the periodic big ones, it isn't always necessary for us to undergo analysis or numb ourselves with drugs in order to cope. For most of us, exercise can do the job.

If we are to prescribe exercise for ourselves, it's important to understand some basic concepts such as aerobic exercise, maximum oxygen uptake, cardiorespiratory fitness, maximum allowable heart rate, and heart rate reserve (defined and discussed in Chapters 2 and 10). With that knowledge, let's begin with some basic guidelines for developing and maintaining fitness and body composition: the recommendations for healthy adults from the American College of Sports Medicine (ACSM).[1] These recommendations concern the quality and quantity of training, specifically spelling out *the kind, frequency, duration, and intensity of exercise necessary to maintain minimal physical fitness.*

The ACSM points out that any kind of activity which (1) involves *large muscle groups*, (2) is *rhythmic*, (3) is *aerobic*, and (4) can be *maintained continuously* will do. Brisk walking, aerobic dancing, running, swimming, skating, bicycling, rowing, and cross-country skiing are common sport activities which fit the ASCM parameters. Working out on a rowing machine, a stationary bicycle, a cross-country ski apparatus, or a treadmill can also fill the bill. These slick-looking chrome-and-black machines appear almost to do the work for us when we see them demonstrated by smiling and fit young men and women. But while they look nice in the ads, they frequently become enemies when we get them home. They are boring, they don't do the work for us, and we rarely smile when using them. I once bought an expensive exercise bike to get me through a running injury. I used it two days and gave it away. You might be the sort of person who can or must come to terms with one of these devices, but you should consider borrowing one and giving it a try for a few weeks before investing your money. If you decide to own one, used ones are, for obvious reasons, very easy to come by.

Whatever it is that we decide to do, ASCM tells us that our exercise must take place *three to five days a week*. Two days does not yield a significant training effect.

The duration of training can vary from *15 to 60 minutes of continuous aerobic activity*. The *duration of exercise periods necessary to yield an increase in cardiorespiratory fitness depends upon the intensity of training*. For healthy nonathletic adults who are just beginning to exercise, activity of moderate intensity and longer duration is best. We are less likely to get discouraged and drop out.

The term *intensity of training* refers to the percentage of our maximum oxygen uptake we must achieve and maintain for the duration of our workout in order to enhance cardiorespiratory fitness. The ASCM tells us that 50 to 85 percent of our maximum oxygen uptake (the greatest volume of oxygen we can take in and effectively deliver to our working muscles in a given period) or 60 to 90 percent of our heart rate reserve is the optimal range to improve cardiorespiratory endurance.

$Vo_{2_{MAX}}$ and HR_{max}

Since few of us can get to an exercise laboratory to be accurately tested for oxygen uptake, we are fortunate that there is a reasonably accurate approximation which we can calculate very easily. Maximum oxygen uptake ($Vo_{2_{MAX}}$) is quite highly correlated with our maximum allowable heart rate (HR_{max}) and *percentage of HR_{max}* can serve our purposes for assessing our personal exercise training intensities. The ASCM training-intensity guideline of *50 to 85 percent of our maximum oxygen uptake corresponds to about 60 to 95 percent of our HR_{max}*.[5]

You will recall that our HR_{max} is related to our age. As we become older our HR_{max} gradually diminishes, and pushing our heart-rate up beyond this limit can be life-threatening. The formula for HR_{max} is 220 minus our age. A 50-year-old woman, for example, would have a HR_{max} of 170 (220 minus 50). A moderate training intensity of 70 percent of her HR_{max} would be about 119 beats per minute, a hard intensity of 80 percent of her HR_{max} would be about 136 beats per minute, and a very hard training intensity of 90 percent of her HR_{max} would be about 161 beats per minute. She should never exceed her 170 HR_{max}.

The older we are, the more out of shape we are, or the more overweight we are, the less is the intensity required to elevate our heart rate to a level where we achieve a training effect and increase our cardiorespiratory fitness.

Taking Our Pulse

Measuring our pulse requires a little care and practice. The best way is to place a couple of fingers over the radial artery of the wrist. The radial artery is on the under side, below the thumb and just inside that knobby bone. It's best to avoid taking a pulse with the thumb as it has a significant artery of its own which can confuse things. Taking a pulse on the carotid artery (the one under our ear and chin bone) can be inaccurate. The carotid artery hates pressure, and the moment we restrict it when taking our pulse, it sends an immediate signal to the brain to dilate the arteries. This quickly lowers our pulse rate. It's wise to learn to do it right and to learn to do it the very moment we stop exercising. Since pulse rate slows quickly when we stop exercising we should take our pulse for only 10 seconds. When we multiply the 10-second reading by 6, we have a measure of our training intensity. Slow down or speed up your pace to get into the desired intensity range, and check it again in a bit. Before long you will know when you are in the ballpark and will seldom have to check.

Pulse rate is a handy thing to know about. We ought to take it every morning. Wake up, grab our watch, lie back down, and relax; then do a 60-second check. Our morning pulse rate is a good gauge of our fitness and lets us know how our training is going. As our training program moves along, our morning resting pulse rate should slowly drop, but it will vary somewhat from day to day. A reading of 10 beats above our average rate on some morning is a signal that something is wrong. It could mean that we are over-training, or it could signal a health problem. It is a definitive warning to cut down the intensity of our training on that day, or better yet, to take the day off.

To Walk or Not to Walk, That Is the Question

The problem with exercise is not so much the getting started as it is the keeping it up. So let's, for the moment, forget about programs, formulas, charts, equipment, costumes, fitness centers, and all of the related commercial hoopla which serves to distract us from the fundamental issue, which is, quite simply, whether or not we exercise.

Epidemiological studies have shown that it doesn't take very much physical activity to make a significant impact on our lives, so long as we do it routinely. The secret is somehow to make exercise an integral part of our lives; something as automatic as getting dressed, eating, and sleeping. It must be something we can do anyplace, anytime, no matter how we are dressed, and without any special equipment.

In the world of exercise, if we seek health and fitness, it basically comes down to whether or not we are willing to walk in a society where walking is no longer necessary. Walking is the foundation, our bedrock life-insurance policy. We may build on it if we choose, but for the most of us it should constitute our basic health plan. There simply isn't anything else that fills the bill. It has to be walking.

Integrating walking into our lives isn't usually all that complicated. While our children might complain, they can often walk to and from school, to the homes of friends, to the movies, and to the record shop. We can walk to work. If our work is a long distance from home, we can park the car two or three miles from work and walk. If we use public transportation, we can get off four or five miles from home in the evening and walk home. Walking home from work allows us some precious time alone to unwind and center ourselves.

We can walk to shop and do our errands. We don't have to buy an entire week's supply of groceries in a single trip. We can buy a few days' supply and walk to the store more frequently. Instead of meeting friends for lunch to discuss how much we need to lose weight, we can meet them for a walk and talk about other, more interesting things. When at work, we can take a long brisk walk at lunchtime.

We can walk around strange cities, in strange countries, and while on hold in airports. In less-than-ideal weather we can walk in covered shopping malls, although these days can often be the most interesting and exhilarating time to be outdoors.

But walking can do more than just get us from one place to another. It can also help us get work done, or it can be a part of our play or recreation. It is a relatively simple thing to say good-bye to our lawn, garden, and pool service, begin to do our own housework and windows, and learn to do considerable home maintenance and home repair. All of these things help us to burn calories through physical activity. Taking care of our own lawns, shrubs, trees, and homes is low-cost cardiac insurance. So is walking the golf course rather than renting a cart.

Walking can buy us added years. The Harvard Alumni Study revealed that walking as few as nine miles a week significantly reduces the likelihood of developing heart disease and reduces the risk of death. The Harvard results suggest that walking 20 to 25 miles a week buys a great deal of protection. That sort of heavy insurance coverage amounts to about an hour of walking four to six days a week. With a very small investment, we can reap significant gains.

Walking has additional benefits. It can reduce the physical tension which comes with daily stresses, help us control our weight, and keep our weight-bearing bones in good shape.

Walking is more convenient than most other forms of physical activity, and it involves no financial risk. If we buy a pair of quality running shoes to begin a walking program, and our intentions fade, we are left with a pair of shoes which are so very comfortable that we may not ever want to wear anything else. Nothing lost except dreams.

Speed, distance, and pulse rates are easy to keep track of when we walk, and walking offers a very safe and simple progression from slow to faster and on to jogging. Walking also lends itself to socializing. Many activities do not.

It's no surprise that walking is becoming more popular in America. This year, for the first time, I have begun to encounter organized club walkers in my favorite mountain running haunts. Some club members come from hundreds of miles to take part in these weekend events. The National Sporting Goods Association tells us that exercise walking has become one of the four most frequently chosen sport activities in America.[6] Sport retailers sold over $5 million worth of walking shoes in 1987, up nearly 40 percent from the previous year. At the same time, running and aerobic dance dropped out of the top 10 activities (if you believe that what people buy is related to what they do).

Walking and Cardiorespiratory Fitness

Walking, it turns out, can be a perfectly adequate training device for most adults. That is to say, almost all of us can increase our cardiorespiratory fitness through walking alone. A most interesting study was done recently at the University of Massachusetts.[5] Several hundred men and women, aged 30 to 69, were simply asked to walk a mile on a flat surface, "as fast as possible." Their pulse rates were measured at the end of the mile walk.

Overall, 67 percent of the men and 91 percent of the women were able to achieve a training intensity of 70 percent of HR_{max} just by being told to walk as fast as they could. The lower percentage of males attaining 70 percent of their HR_{max} was explained by the fact that the men in the 30 to 59 age group were already very physically fit, approaching Dr. Ken Cooper's "high fit" category.

For the older men and women (50 to 69 years of age), 83 percent of the men and 91 percent of the women attained 70 percent of HR_{max}.

Some very highly fit young men had difficulty in achieving 70 percent HR_{max} when simply told to walk as fast as possible, but when informed of their target heart-rate, and provided with constant heart-rate visual feedback, all were able to attain the desired training intensity while walking very briskly for a 25-minute period.

The figures for the various groups are encouraging in that they make it clear that it is easier to attain a fitness-enhancing intensity if we are either older or more out of shape to begin with. If we unfit adults are going to begin a walking program, it is a good idea to train at a moderate intensity (60 to 70 percent of HR_{max}) for a couple of months. Some of us who remain very overweight or who are older may choose never to exceed moderate training intensities.

Figuring out our moderate training range is very simple. HR_{max} (220 minus our age) times .60, and then times .70, gives us our personal moderate-training-intensity heartbeat range. A moderate range for a 40-year-old works out to 108 to 126 heartbeats per minute, while that of a 30-year-old works out to 114 to 133 beats per minute. Knowledge of our target heart-rate range allows us to pursue increased fitness using any form of exercise which fits the four ACSM criteria.

Using Exercise Time Effectively

While walking might provide all of the fitness many of us desire, there are some advantages to increasing the intensity of our training. The ACSM points out that, for adequate fitness, we must train at 50 to 85 percent of our maximum oxygen uptake for from 15 to 60 minutes, three to five times a week. These wide parameters suggest that, if we exercise at higher intensities, we can get all of the fitness we want in less time, and on fewer days. Thus, by moving from a walking phase to a walk-jog phase, and on to a jogging-only phase, we can save considerable time.

New research now demonstrates that we can increase our maximum oxygen uptake substantially by working out as little as 12 minutes three times a week by doing interval training.[4] I'll discuss interval training in a moment, but first a cautionary note. Faster and more efficient isn't always better, particularly for those of us who are already caught up in Type A behavior patterns. A good, hard half-hour workout three times a week is about all some of us can afford, but if exercise becomes just one more frantic activity in an already frantic life, we might take pause and consider the quality of our existence and what it all means.

Exercise to Increase Fitness and Cardiac Reserve

There are many sound reasons for us to increase our cardiorespiratory fitness beyond minimal levels. Some of us might want to increase it in order to compete in our chosen sport, or to build endurance for another sport. Boxers, skiers, and tennis players, for example, frequently engage in distance running several days each week.

Perhaps our goal is to achieve more substantial cardiac reserve or significantly reduced heart-attack risk. If our family history is one of deaths from coronary heart disease, and if our cholesterol counts underline our risk, we might want to make a very large investment in regular exercise of substantial quality and quantity in order to compensate for our above-average risk of coronary heart disease. You will recall that the aerobic equivalent of at least 10 miles of jogging each week appears to be necessary in order to elevate the levels of the "good" HDL cholesterol in our blood plasma. Exercising with greater intensity, duration, and frequency also provides heart-rate reserve which could help us to survive severe stress.

If we wish to become faster swimmers, bicyclists, or runners, it's necessary to train appropriately for speed. Such training involves "interval work," which translates into introducing intervals or bursts of very intense effort into our training. For example, after warming up, instead of running at a constant pace, we might alternate sprinting for one minute with two minutes of slow jogging several times during a half-hour run. We can easily translate this into bicycling, working on a rowing machine, or swimming by applying the same basic principles of intervals of increased and decreased intensity. Aerobic-dance teachers are beginning to introduce interval work into their training routines. Interval training provides a substantial payoff, but involves the usual risks that come along with big, fast gains.

The payoff is dramatic increases in aerobic capacity (maximum oxygen uptake), more rapid increases than those achieved with the sort of steady training recommended a decade ago when the ACSM set up its criteria. Many recent studies now consistently show that interval training can rapidly enhance cardiorespiratory fitness. The risks associated with interval training center on injury.

It is much easier to hurt ourselves while doing bursts of highly strenuous interval work than while doing regular, steady training. When doing interval work we should always be warmed up. What's more, we should not make it a daily routine. While a little can be good, more can become a nightmare.

Another important consideration is that while interval training may give us dramatic, rapid gains in cardiorespiratory fitness, it doesn't provide us with everything we might wish for. Training is a very specific sort of activity with very specific outcomes. If we want to be fast, we must train fast (do interval speed work). If we want to possess the capacity for great endurance, we must do endurance training (long and steady workouts). If we want both, we must do both. We might, for example, do interval work one or two days a week, and endurance training three or more days a week.

Exercise to Control Mood

Another reason for deciding to increase our training intensity has to do with mood control. While walking can provide many of the things which running can deliver, we don't know whether it offers the relief from depression which running provides. Walking may very well have the potential to reduce depression, but it may have to be very brisk walking, the sort which provides a training effect.

While there is no definitive answer to this question, there is considerable encouraging testimony from sedentary individuals who have taken up walking. Each semester I have a number of people enrolled in my class on exercise and mental health who decide to begin to walk briskly an hour each day in order to lose weight. They don't ordinarily tell me about this until the semester is over and they can tell me about the pounds they have shed. They then report that the daily one-hour walks not only helped them to lose weight but also elevated their moods. While this is only testimony, it is consistent and does suggest that brisk walking may have the potential to elevate moods.

The research we have reviewed in this book consistently shows that 30 minutes of aerobic exercise three times a week will significantly reduce depression. For many of us three such sessions of aerobic dance, jogging, swimming, or working out on an exercise machine might be sufficient to deal with a period of depression. Other research suggests that the antidepressant effects of exercise are acute, lasting only 12 to 26 hours. This finding suggests that for some of us, more than three workouts each week may be necessary to deal with a substantial depression. While exercise has immediate or acute antidepressant effects, research suggests that significant reduction in depressive symptoms takes place in three to five weeks. Daily exercise could also have a prophylactic effect, protecting us from the mood depressions which we would ordinarily experience.

Exercise to Control Anxiety

Exercise can also produce a very significant tranquilizing effect which can help us to deal with the periods of anxiety which periodically trouble us. The tranquilizing effects of exercise appear to be far more acute than its antidepressant effects, lasting for a matter of about 2 to 4 hours. Thus, exercise might be thought of as a tool we can bring into play when we suffer an anxious period, rather than as something which will forever keep our anxiety at bay. There is some question about the intensity of exercise which is required to reduce anxiety. Physiological state anxiety (which is importantly reflected in muscle tension) can be reduced by 5 to 30 minutes of very-low-intensity (30 percent to 60 percent of maximum oxygen uptake) rhythmic exercise such as walking, jogging, or cycling. But research on psychological state anxiety (which is reflected by psychological tests that assess how much anxiety we are experiencing) suggests that exercise of a greater intensity (70 percent of maximum oxygen uptake) than that typically provided by walking is required for significant anxiety reductions. On the other hand, a variety of distracting activities such as meditation or simply taking "time out" can also effectively reduce psychological state anxiety.

All of this would suggest that almost any form of exercise might be effective, depending on the cause and intensity of our anxiety. If very moderate exercise doesn't do the job, then perhaps a more vigorous workout will. A long, brisk walk might relax our muscles, but a tough aerobic-dance workout might be required to distract us and reduce the psychological anxiety we are experiencing.

Men and women who exercise daily to deal with stress learn to schedule a workout when they most need it. Some find a morning workout helps get them through the tough part of the day, others work out at lunchtime to best cope with tension on the job, and still others work out at night to shed the tension accumulated through the day. Others of us who live relatively unstressful lives may utilize exercise to deal with anxiety on an "as-needed" basis. The frequency and intensity of exercise required to cope with our anxiety and stress will vary, depending on the cause, intensity, and duration of our stressors. Whatever the case, exercise provides a good alternative to tranquilizing drugs.

Men and women who run rate the postrun "afterglow" as one of the primary reasons for regular workouts. The rather marvelously tranquil and relaxed state which routinely follows each session of exercise may not be something that we are willing to think of only as an "as-needed" intervention when we are feeling unusually anxious. Once we get a taste for it, many of us are unwilling to let a day pass without experiencing those delicious hours of afterglow.

Exercise for Weight Control

Whether we walk, run, swim, bicycle, or combine several physical activities, it is wise to keep our goals in mind. While cardiorespiratory fitness and relief from depression can be achieved with a few moderately intense workouts each week, many of us are also concerned about weight control.

Sensible weight control demands daily activity, and the most efficient way to burn off calories is with sustained moderate exercise. If we exercise strenuously three times a week for cardiorespiratory fitness, such exercise should be considered a supplement to periods of moderate, sustained exercise for weight control.[2]

In Chapter 10 we saw how our body utilizes fat as a fuel at an increasing rate as our exercise continues over a sustained time period, how regular bouts of extended exercise will shape our physiology so that we become more efficient fat-burners, and how exercise should be central in a weight control program.

If we are very strongly motivated to lose weight, a first priority would be to organize our lives in such a way that we have a full hour free each day for exercise. If we have previously been sedentary, we might begin with an hour of walking each day, and as we gradually become more fit and shed some pounds, we could increase our speed and distance. Eventually we might jog a little. The key to shedding pounds through exercise is to work out each day for a substantial time period at a moderate intensity. When we have lost the pounds we wish to be rid of and have increased our fitness, we can think of modifying our exercise program.

If this sounds like an enormous or even heroic undertaking, it may help to realize that others have felt as you do. You might begin by talking to friends who have incorporated regular exercise into their lives. You may discover that they no longer see exercise as a negative chore. They wouldn't keep it up if it didn't make them feel good and make them feel good about themselves. You've got to figure that once established, regular exercise must be self-sustaining and that the rewards must importantly overshadow whatever inconveniences or problems such a lifestyle change brings.

Choosing Exercise We Can Live With

If our exercise program is going to endure, it is critical that we choose exercise we can live with. Recall the story of my friend who coached the alpine ski team. The high boredom susceptibility of many sensation seekers, such as downhill ski racers, doomed his jogging prescription from the start.[7]

For those of us who are easily bored, there are a number of options. One is to engage in different activities on different days of the week. We might get our cardiovascular conditioning with three aerobic-dance days, then walk, swim, or bicycle for weight control on others. Some of us need the challenge of competition to hold our interest. Tennis, volleyball, basketball, and racquetball are all options. Singles tennis and doubles volleyball obviously offer a more strenuous workout than do doubles tennis or regular six-person volleyball.

Brooklyn College professor Dr. Bonnie Berger suggests that there are many factors which can importantly influence what sort of sport or exercise we are likely to chose and stick with.[3] She lists the predictability of the sport environment, the probability of physical harm, and the directness of competition as playing significant roles, pointing out that the predictable environments of sports such as distance swimming or running allow us to tune into our own thoughts, while the unpredictable environment of a basketball or tennis court requires intense attention focus, the sort of thing which might serve to distract us from our worries and concerns. These different sports contain other significant and sometimes unique social aspects which can be importantly related to our needs. If we want to make a physical activity a part of our lives, it is wise to consider our individual needs beyond simply our desire to become more fit.

Where we live can also be an important determiner in setting up a program of exercise. Living near a gym, a year-round swimming pool, a mountain fire trail, a ski area, country roads, the beach, or a park can importantly influence what we will do and how long we are likely to keep it up. It's very important to choose activities which are convenient.

Fun can also enter in. Other things being equal, we are more likely to keep on exercising if we are having a good time. If feasible, it makes good sense to go back to a sport or activity which we enjoyed in the past. The odds are we will still find pleasure in it for the same reason as in the past. If it's impossible or impractical to renew our friendship with an old sport, perhaps there is something new that looks good to us. Maybe we have a friend who is doing something we would like to try. People who exercise are usually willing to help others get started.

Exercise and Companionship

Committing ourselves to exercise daily with a friend can have a powerful reinforcing effect. One of the very best ways to get started on exercise and to maintain it is to make a regular date with

a friend. A walk is ideal in almost all respects. It offers companionship, incentive to keep up the routine, and encouragement when
we need it. There are days when we just don't feel like exercising.
We may feel depressed, deenergized, harried, or as if we may be
becoming ill. If a friend can get us out of the house and physically
active, we soon learn that the times we least feel like exercising are
the most rewarding times to do it. Morning walks can prepare us
for the day. Morning seems to be the time preferred by the many
women I encounter on my running routes. Weekends are good
times for very long hikes or bicycle rides with members of our
family or friends.

I like companionship when I set out on longer runs in the
mountains. Having someone to talk with makes the miles drift by
quite magically. I have also discovered that when running marathons, chatting with people has always helped distract me from
the inevitable physical pain which comes after hours of running.
Teaming up with someone is always a simple matter. I recall running a dreadfully hot marathon one summer, and teaming up with
a young girl of about 10 or 12. Her father's early pace was a little
too much for her, and our pace seemed about right for 15 miles or
so, until she took off and left me behind. Whether we are walking
with a friend in the neighborhood or running a marathon with
people we have never before met, a rewarding part of the activity is
that we always seem to be doing something with someone rather
than against someone.

Team sports can also offer a marvelous sort of camaraderie and
support. Soccer, basketball, and hockey are not only social and fun
but can also enhance cardiorespiratory conditioning. If we need
social contact, adult league team sports might fill the bill. Competitive sports can also serve to distract us from the stresses of our lives
in a way that few other activities can. For some of us competition
and camaraderie are necessary ingredients if we are to exercise at
all. For others, however, competition is a virtual guarantee of
nonparticipation.

If our lives are overflowing with people and their demands,
our exercise time might be our personal time for solitude. A solo
walk, swim, or bike ride might provide the essential peace of mind.
I received a letter from a runner in Indiana which conveys a familiar theme. He wrote as follows:

I'm 54 years old now, and 35 of those years have been used raising and educating children, paying for a home, and all of the other things that are required of a husband and a father. There was no time left to think for myself. Running is the one thing that I do for myself and myself alone.

Thus, who we are and the nature of our daily lives importantly dictate what sort of physical activity is likely to fit our needs, and it has to make sense to no one other than ourselves.

Getting Started

If our exercise plans involve more than simply incorporating walking into our daily lifestyles, and we wish to begin a program for increased fitness and weight control, here are some guidelines on how to get started. Let's talk in terms of walking, but bear in mind that what I have to say can be translated into most other kinds of aerobic activities.

It makes sense to set up an initial goal, either a time or a distance which we wish to walk each session. These goals should be modest and flexible. We can always extend or modify them as we discover how our motivation and physical condition interact and react to exercise.

The typical exercise program which has been so consistently used by researchers who have investigated the role of exercise in the reduction of depression goes something like this. Three 45- to 50-minute sessions are scheduled on alternate days during each week. Individuals stretch and warm up for 10 minutes before and following a 30-minute walk-jog session. Walking and jogging are alternated. At first, most of the time is spent walking, with only short periods of jogging, but as the weeks go by, jogging takes an increasing proportion of the time. Most of us can eventually jog for the full 30-minute session, usually covering somewhere between 2½ and 3½ miles. Depending on our age, weight, and condition, this could take a matter of a month or two, or as long as a year.

Some of us might then continue to jog for a half hour three times a week and gradually increase the distance we cover during that time period. Others might decide to increase the frequency of their 30-minute runs up to four or five times each week or to increase their jogging time to 45 minutes or an hour three times a week. There are all sorts of options once we are able to run for 30 minutes. We might even decide to enter a five-kilometer race and meet our unknown brothers and sisters.

Instead of exercising for a given time period, another option is to chose a given distance. Here is a letter I received from a 53-year-old woman from Washington, D.C. While she has now run more than 8000 miles, she wrote of her first mile and how she began to run for certain reasons, but continued because of unanticipated rewards:

> I started to run because I was flabby and out of shape. I kept on running because I liked the way it made me feel. I had never dreamed that I could run a mile. Women of my generation were never encouraged to think of themselves as potential athletes. All of the thousands of miles I have run have never given me the thrill of my first mile. It took me five months of training to finally do it, and I will never forget it. I'll be running the rest of my life, God willing.

The time-distance formula can be adjusted to any activity. Swimming pools offer laps for computing distance or for alternating easy and more strenuous efforts. Bicycling is a little tougher unless you live in an area where there are trails or roads which are free of traffic and stoplights. A bicycle odometer is cheap, and it is an easy matter to identify landmarks which serve to mark mileage.

Bicycling, running, and walking all offer their own forms of interval training if we live in an area where there are hills. Working extra hard on the uphills can boost our fitness very significantly. Hills are also less boring for our muscle groups when we are walking or running.

Our bodies are so marvelously plastic and have the capacity to adapt to what we ask of them. Our cardiovascular age can be almost whatever we shape it to be. It is very difficult to know just exactly what our limits are—and what our ultimate lifestyle will be like—when we begin a modest exercise program. Here is a letter from a woman who has now run more than 30,000 miles. She summarizes her motives for running:

> For the first 57 years of my life I was a daughter, student, member of the military, mother, student a second time, grandmother, and a librarian. Then I broke my collarbone in a bicycle accident. I took a weight-lifting class to strengthen my shoulder. The course included a lap around the track, and I found that I couldn't do a single lap. I

looked in the mirror and saw a fat old woman. I didn't like her. I work on a university campus where a few people run instead of sitting and eating at lunchtime. I joined them. That was seven years ago. Now I love my running and I love the new me—the me that was hidden all those years has emerged, 30 pounds lighter and with the heart and lungs of a 20-year-old (my doctor said so last week). I am not fond of doing intervals, but I visit the track once a week. Mostly I run the back roads and trails in the Santa Cruz Mountains, either alone or with a friend. I run every day, hate the heat, and love the cold and rain. Very early mornings are the best.

This woman may seem extraordinary to the 80 percent of us in the United States who are just plain unfit. Our primary goal is simply to exercise. So forget the stopwatch, mileage, pulse, and caloric burn rate. Just get moving.

Whether one is an experienced athlete or a beginner, the problem frequently comes down the taking that first step each day. Even though I have been running almost daily now and have run more than 16,000 miles over the last decade, some mornings it seems next to impossible to get started. I find myself standing and shivering on cold mornings down at the end of my driveway, unwilling to take that first step. My neighbors drive by in warm cars, shaking their heads and wondering when I am going to begin to act my age.

I know that I will eventually lean forward and be forced to take that first step to keep from falling on my face. I also know that the rewards when I am done will make me grateful I did it, but that first step can be tough on some days. What's even worse is that sometimes the running itself feels awful for the first mile or so. But I have learned over the years that if I can take the first step, the rest of the steps will take care of themselves.

This lesson in faith which I continue to affirm at the bottom of my driveway has carried me though some brutal marathons and took me up what seemed like an impossible long and steep ice face at 20,000 feet on the border of Tibet a couple of years ago. So whether its crampons and ice axes or lacing on sneakers before a marathon, I have learned that what seems like the impossible can be dealt with on a one-step-at-a-time basis. If we know that, the first step is the key. After that we can deal with the steps which follow. Yesterday is gone. The future is yet to be. It is only today and this single step.

Staying Healthy and Alive

Steps taken toward a healthier, happier life should be taken with both enthusiasm and care. It is wise to consult with a physician before we embark on an exercise program. Sometimes, for example, exercise can affect conditions for which we're taking medication. We might also have a special physical condition which may put us at risk and can exercise safely only with medical supervision. Earlier chapters have discussed an number of specific issues which relate to risks associated with exercise, but let me share some general guidelines which might be helpful in keeping healthy and injury-free.

Most experts suggest warm-up (down) and stretching both prior to and after exercising. Some forms of exercise allow us to warm up by beginning the exercise at a very moderate level. For example, I always use the first mile of running as a warm-up and do all of my stretching after the run at a time when my muscles are warm and flexible. Many of my friends follow the same routine (after we injured ourselves by stretching when cold prior to running). Regardless of the nature of the warm-up, it should be cautious and moderate.

Without question, the single most important fundamental rule concerning all aspects of an exercise program is moderation. We are going to hurt ourselves if we do too much too fast. Once we discover that we can do something which previously seemed impossible, such as running or swimming an entire mile, it's so very easy to become overly enthusiastic and overdo it. While one day of interval training each week might produce a remarkable increase in speed, three days a week might bring us injury and months of no exercise at all.

We should increase the intensity, duration, and frequency of our workouts in very small increments. A common guideline is the rule of "no more than 10 percent increase a week." Thus, if we have run 10 miles in a week for the first time, 11 miles the following week is a sensible goal, one which will probably keep us running rather than necessitating a trip to the drugstore to purchase ice packs and elastic bandages.

It's tough to behave with moderation in the full bloom of early enthusiasm. It's even tougher to let an injury heal properly once we have done the damage. A large number of the injuries we incur are caused by overuse, and the very motives which prompted us to do too much make it very hard to stop our preferred mode of exercising. The second rule is to *give our injuries time to heal*. We should believe the doctor, and not go from one specialist to another, hoping one will give us the pill, the shot, the bandage, the ultrasound, the special magic to make it somehow all right for us to continue exercising while we are injured. *If it hurts, don't use it.* Almost all overuse injuries will heal very nicely on their own if we give them time. Sometimes a physician can recommend an alternative form of exercise which will keep us fit until our injury heals and we can get back to doing our favorite thing. Most of us at one time or another overdo it and hurt ourselves, and most of us will at some point refuse to allow an injury to heal properly before further damaging ourselves. If we are lucky, we survive these early mistakes and learn.

So the basic guidelines are to warm up and warm down; to use moderation when increasing duration, intensity, and frequency of exercise; and to allow our injuries the time to heal properly.

Walt Stack, a well-known San Francisco runner who carries bricks for a living, has a very simple guideline for racing. A decade or so ago I sometimes chatted with him during marathons. I think he was about 70 then, and was already a legendary figure. Walt always took a morning dip in the bay before running a 17-mile route across the Golden Gate Bridge and back. The run was followed by a second dip in the freezing bay waters. He then carried bricks for eight hours.

Walt runs races with a personal philosophy which keeps him smiling and agreeable to having an occasional beer as he jogs for four or five hours through a marathon. It's a philosophy which has served him well. He says that his secret is to "Start slow, and then taper off."

Epilogue

This book suggests that we Americans have lost our way during this century. Our experiment with a seductive lifestyle, contrary to the one we lived for all but this final moment of our evolution, has been a costly one.

After 50,000 years, we suddenly changed our diets, learned to smoke, and became sedentary. We began to die prematurely from a variety of chronic diseases which reflected our new ways of living, and we began to suffer high rates of depression and anxiety disorders. Many of us turned to alcohol and drugs to ease our troubled minds.

While many features of our stress-filled contemporary life contribute to the anxiety and depression which so many of us suffer, I have suggested that our unnatural sedentary ways have played a role. By becoming physically inactive we have lost the daily tranquilizing and mood-elevating effects which exercise provides. Those of us who live sedentary lifestyles are, in a sense, unnaturally depressed and anxious.

Depression is a major mental-health problem in America, and with the exception of the bipolar disorders, exercise appears to be an effective treatment. Exercise therapy appears to be as powerful as antidepressant drugs and the psychotherapies, and it offers many strengths and advantages which those more conventional treatments do not offer. It's side effects are beneficent and life-enhancing.

Exercise can serve as a primary treatment for our normal depressions as well as for depressions which are the result of moderate biochemical systemic imbalances. When depression is the result of maladaptive behavior patterns, exercise can serve as an adjunctive treatment to psychotherapy. Exercise has an immediate acute effect, elevating mood for as long as a full day in both normal and severely depressed individuals. Clinically depressed individuals who begin to exercise regularly are usually symptom-free in about three weeks.

Exercise also has an acute anxiety-reducing effect which will last for several hours. It can be scheduled into our lives to deal with predictable daily stresses or it can be used on an "as-needed" basis to deal with periodic crises. Thus, exercise can be used to reduce the depression and anxiety associated with events which have just occurred, or it can be used to minimize the effects of stresses which are expected. Regular daily exercise can do both.

Regular physical activity yields a vast array of positive consequences and must have been a central component in our evolutionary blueprinting. We evolved as active creatures, and we just don't seem to work well or feel good without regular physical activity. Sedentary life is a violation of our genetic warranty.

We don't have to turn our backs on all of the wondrous benefits of civilization to reclaim the essential life-enhancing aspects of our old hunter-gatherer ways. Becoming physically active, stopping smoking, and going back to diets more akin to those of our ancestors is all that is required. If we embraced these old ways and lived as we were designed to live in this age of sanitation and modern medicine, we would redefine normality and rewrite what it means to act our age. Throughout our lifetime we would have strong muscles, bones, and cardiovascular systems. We would remain flexible and lean and would maintain both physical and mental vitality. Visits to physicians and lost workdays would be few. We would experience less anxiety and depression and would be better equipped to deal with stress. We can add years to our life, and life to our years. The choices are ours. What a fortunate time to be alive, and what splendiferous choices.

Appendix

Test of Endurance Athlete Motives (TEAM)

This test is designed to measure the relative strength of the most common motives for regular exercise or endurance training. The motives which impel us to begin to exercise may change in strength over time, so it is important to take this test with a specific time frame in mind, either as a measure of *current motives* or as a retrospective measure of your *initial motives* when you first began to exercise or train regularly. You may wish to take the test twice to assess both initial and current motives.

The test involves making forced choices between pairs of motives which are listed on the next page. Each motive is paired once with each other motive, and you must *select the one of the two alternatives which is most important to you* and mark the appropriate square. Even if both alternatives of a given pair are of little importance to you, it is important that you select one of them so that the test can be properly scored. The motivation test form does not include the motive "Fame and Fortune." If this motive has more relevance to your life than "Addictions," please substitute it for "Addictions" on the Motivation Test Form.

The test is scored by simply adding up the number of times each motive was selected. No motive can have a score greater than 9, and the total of your 10 scores must be 45. This paired-comparison format yields scores which reflect the relative strength of the motives included.

Motive Definitions

Addictions: To stop or control antilife habits such as smoking, drinking, or drug use through regular exercise.

Afterglow: The elevated mood and reduced tension which follow regular exercise.

Centering: Space to be alone, to clear my head, and to simply experience myself and the world around me. The psychological experience while exercising.

Challenge: To challenge or gradually improve myself through participation. To perform better than I did in the past.

Compete: To challenge others and to define myself in relation to other competitors.

Fame and Fortune: To make money and/or a name for myself as an athlete.

Feels Good: The various rewarding physical experiences while exercising; the exercise itself feels good to me.

Fitness: The cardiovascular and general physical fitness which follows regular exercise.

Identity: The independent definition of or statement about myself: I exercise. I am an athlete. It is my lifestyle.

Slim: To control weight and appetite through regular exercise.

Social: To meet new friends or to be with old ones through exercise, competition, or club activities.

MOTIVATION TEST FORM

☐ FITNESS ☐ FEELS GOOD	☐ SLIM ☐ COMPETE	☐ AFTERGLOW ☐ FEELS GOOD	☐ ADDICTIONS ☐ FITNESS	☐ IDENTITY ☐ CENTERING
☐ CENTERING ☐ FITNESS	☐ FITNESS ☐ IDENTITY	☐ COMPETE ☐ CENTERING	☐ SOCIAL ☐ FITNESS	☐ IDENTITY ☐ SLIM
☐ ADDICTIONS ☐ FEELS GOOD	☐ SOCIAL ☐ SLIM	☐ FITNESS ☐ AFTERGLOW	☐ IDENTITY ☐ CHALLENGE	☐ COMPETE ☐ ADDICTIONS
☐ ADDICTIONS ☐ SOCIAL	☐ IDENTITY ☐ AFTERGLOW	☐ SLIM ☐ CHALLENGE	☐ CENTERING ☐ SOCIAL	☐ FITNESS ☐ COMPETE
☐ CHALLENGE ☐ CENTERING	☐ CENTERING ☐ AFTERGLOW	☐ SLIM ☐ CENTERING	☐ FEELS GOOD ☐ SOCIAL	☐ IDENTITY ☐ ADDICTIONS
☐ COMPETE ☐ SOCIAL	☐ AFTERGLOW ☐ ADDICTIONS	☐ SOCIAL ☐ AFTERGLOW	☐ SLIM ☐ AFTERGLOW	☐ CHALLENGE ☐ ADDICTIONS
☐ ADDICTIONS ☐ CENTERING	☐ FEELS GOOD ☐ COMPETE	☐ FITNESS ☐ CHALLENGE	☐ COMPETE ☐ IDENTITY	☐ CHALLENGE ☐ FEELS GOOD
☐ SLIM ☐ FEELS GOOD	☐ CHALLENGE ☐ SOCIAL	☐ ADDICTIONS ☐ SLIM	☐ IDENTITY ☐ SOCIAL	☐ AFTERGLOW ☐ CHALLENGE
☐ CENTERING ☐ FEELS GOOD	☐ IDENTITY ☐ FEELS GOOD	☐ COMPETE ☐ CHALLENGE	☐ SLIM ☐ FITNESS	☐ AFTERGLOW ☐ COMPETE

References

CHAPTER 1

1. Bule, J. (1983, October). "Me" decades generate depression. *APA Monitor*, p. 18.
2. Egeland, J. A., Gerhard, D. S., Pauls, D. L., *et al.* (1987). Bipolar affective disorders linked to DNA markers on chromosome 11. *Nature, 325,* 783–787.
3. Feist, J., & Brannon, L. (1988). *Health Psychology.* Belmont, CA: Wadsworth.
4. Fries, J. F., & Crapo, L. M. (1981). *Vitality and Aging.* San Francisco: Freeman.
5. Hayflick, L. (1980). The cell biology of human aging. *Scientific American, 242,* 58–65.
6. Kirschenbaum, D. S. (1987). Toward the prevention of sedentary lifestyles. In W. P. Morgan & S. E. Goldston (Eds.), *Exercise and Mental Health* (pp. 17–35). Washington, DC: Hemisphere.
7. Leaf, A. (1973). Unusual longevity—The common denominator. *Hospital Practice, 8,* 75–86.
8. Murphy, J. M., Sobol, A. M., Neff, R. K., *et al.* (1984). Stability of prevalence: Depression and anxiety disorders. *Archives of General Psychiatry, 41,* 990–997.
9. Myers, J. K., Weissman, M. M., Tischler, G. L., *et al.* (1984). Six-month prevalence of psychiatric disorders in three communities. *Archives of General Psychiatry, 41,* 959–967.
10. Robins, L. N., Helzer, J. E., Weissman, M. M., *et al.* (1984). Lifetime prevalence of specific psychiatric disorder in three sites. *Archives of General Psychiatry, 41,* 949–958.
11. Sime, W. E. (1987). Exercise in the prevention and treatment of depression. In W. P. Morgan & S. E. Goldston (Eds.), *Exercise and Mental Health,* (pp. 145–152). Washington, DC: Hemisphere.

CHAPTER 2

1. Carmack, M. A., & Martens, R. (1979). Measuring commitment to running: A survey of runner's attitudes and mental states. *Journal of Sports Psychology, 1,* 25–42.
2. Edmiston, B. (1984). *The Motivation of Women Distance Runners and Aerobic Dancers.* Unpublished senior paper, San Jose State University, Department of Psychology.
3. Johnsgård, K. (1981, July). You're never too old. *Runner's World,* pp. 70–75.
4. Johnsgård, K. (1985). The motivation of the long-distance runner: I. *Journal of Sports Medicine and Physical Fitness, 25*(3), 135–139.
5. Johnsgård, K. (1985). The motivation of the long-distance runner: II. *Journal of Sports Medicine and Physical Fitness, 25*(3), 140–143.
6. Johnsgård, K., & Suggs, E. (1985, May). Why we do it: A psychological study of *Running Times* readers. *Running Times,* pp. 22–25.
7. Zuckerman, M. (1979). *Sensation Seeking: Beyond the Optimal Level of Arousal.* Hillsdale, NJ: Erlbaum.
8. Zuckerman, M. (Ed.). (1983). *Biological Bases of Sensation Seeking, Impulsivity, and Anxiety.* Hillsdale, NJ: Erlbaum.

CHAPTER 3

1. Allen, M. G. (1976). Twin studies in affective illness. *Archives of General Psychiatry, 33,* 1476–1478.
2. Åsberg, M., Thoren, P., Traskman, L., et al. (1972). Serotonin depression—A biochemical subgroup within the affective disorders? *Science, 191,* 478–480.
3. Bourne, H. R., Bunney, W. E., Colburn, R. W., et al. (1968, October 12). Noradrenaline, 5-hydroxytryptamine and 5-hydroxyindoleacetic acid in hindbrains of suicidal patients. *Lancet,* pp. 805–808.
4. Bridgeman, B. (1988). *The Biology of Behavior and Mind.* New York: Wiley.
5. Brown, G. L., Goodwin, J. C., Ballinger, P. F., et al. (1979). Aggression in human correlates with cerebrospinal fluid amine metabolites. *Psychiatry Research, 1,* 131–139.
6. Bule, J. (1983, October). "Me" decades generate depression. *APA Monitor,* p. 18.
7. Creese, I., Burt, D. R., & Snyder, S. H. (1976). Dopamine receptor binding predicts clinical and pharmacological potencies of antischizophrenic drugs. *Science, 192,* 481– 483.
8. *Diagnostic and Statistical Manual of Mental Disorders (DSM-III).* (1980). Washington, DC: American Psychiatric Association.
9. Egeland, J. A., Gerhard, D. S., Pauls, D. L., et al. (1987). Bipolar affective disorders linked to DNA markers on chromosome 11. *Nature, 325,* 783–787.
10. Fishman, S. M., & Sheehan, D. V. (1985, April). Anxiety and panic: Their cause and treatment. *Psychology Today,* pp. 26–31.
11. Fowler, C. J., von Knorring, L., & Oreland, L. (1980). Platelet monoamine oxidase activity in sensation seekers. *Psychiatry Research, 3,* 273–279.

12. Garver, D. L., & Davis, J. M. (1979). Minireview: Biogenic amine hyptheses of affective disorders. *Life Sciences, 24,* 383–394.
13. Hopson, J. L. (1988, July/August). A pleasureable chemistry. *Psychology Today,* pp. 29–33.
14. Janowsky, D., El-Yousef, M., Davis, J., & Sekerke, H. (1982). Parasympathetic suppression of manic symptoms by physostigmine. *Archives of General Psychiatry, 139,* 1162–1164.
15. Kennedy, J., Giuffra, L., Moises, H., *et al.* (1988, November 10). Evidence against linkage of schizophrenia to markers on chromosome 5 in a northern Swedish pedigree. *Nature, 336,* 167–170.
16. Lander, E. S. (1988, November 10). Splitting schizophrenia. *Nature, 336,* 105–106.
17. Lee, T., & Seeman, P. (1980). Elevation of brain neuroleptic/dopamine receptors in schizophrenia. *American Journal of Psychiatry, 137,* 191–197.
18. Linnoila, M., Virkkunen, M., Scheinin, M., *et al.* (1983). Low cerebrospinal fluid 5-hydroxyindoleacetic acid concentration differentiates impulsive for nonimpulsive violent behavior. *Life Science, 23,* 2609–2614.
19. Mann, J. J., McBride, P. A., & Stanley, M. (1986). Postmortem monoamine receptor and enzyme studies in suicide. *Annals New York Academy of Sciences, 487,* 114–121.
20. Murphy, J. M., Sobol, A. M., Neff, R. K., *et al.* (1984). Stabilty of prevalence: Depression and anxiety disorders. *Archives of General Psychiatry, 41,* 990–997.
21. Myers, J. K., Weissman, M. M., Tischler, G. L., *et al.* (1984). Six-month prevalence of psychiatric disorders in three communities. *Archives of General Psychiatry, 41,* 959-967.
22. Nardi, N., Nurnberger, J., Jr., & Gershon, E. (1984). Muscarinic cholinergic receptors in skin fibroblasts in familial affective disorders. *New England Journal of Medicine, 311,* 225–230.
23. Nurnberger, J. I. & Gershon, E. S. (1982). Genetics. In E. S. Paykel (Ed.), *Handbook of Affective Disorders.* New York: Guilford Press.
24. Perse, T. (1988). Obsessive-compulsive disorder: A treatment review. *Journal of Clinical Psychiatry, 49*(2), 48–55.
25. Regier, D. A., Meyers, J. K., Kramer, M., *et al.* (1984). The NIMH epidemiologic catchment area program. *Archives of General Psychiatry, 41,* 934–941.
26. Robins, L. N., Helzer, J. E., Weissman, M. M., *et al.* (1984). Lifetime prevalence of specific psychiatric disorder in three sites. *Archives of General Psychiatry, 41,* 949–958.
27. Secunda, S. K., Cross, C. K., Koslow, S, *et al.* (1986). Studies of amine metabolites in depressed patients. *Annals of New York Academy of Sciences, 487,* 231–241.
28. Shapiro, S., Skinner, E. A., Kessler, L. G., *et al.* (1984). Utilization of health and mental health services: Three epidemiologic catchment area sites. *Archives of General Psychiatry, 41,* 971–978.
29. Sherrington, R., Brynjolfsson, J., Pettursson, H., *et al.* (1988, November 10). Localization of a susceptibility locus for schizophrenia on chromosome 5. *Nature, 336,* 164–167.
30. Snyder, S. H. (1980). *Biological Aspects of Mental Disorder.* New York: Oxford.

31. Snyder, S. H. (1984). Cholinergic mechanisms in affective disorders. *New England Journal of Medicine, 311*, 254.
32. Stanford scientists find possible clue to autism. (1985, February 11). *San Jose Mercury News*.
33. Stewart, A. L., & Brook, R. H. (1983). Effects of being overweight. *American Journal of Public Health, 73*(2), 171–178.
34. Talan, J. (1986, November 15). Sober pill for addicts? *San Jose Mercury News*, pp. 1–2C.
35. Taube, C. A., Burns, B. J., & Kessler, L. (1984). Patients of psychiatrists and psychologists in office-based practice: 1980. *American Psychologist, 39*(12), 1435–1447.
36. Twenty two percent were molested as kids, poll says. (1985, August 25). *San Jose Mercury News*.
37. Wetterberg, L. (1982). The genetic control of catecholamines and its possible implication in schizophrenia. In G. Hemmings (Ed.), *Biological Aspects of Schizophrenia and Addiction*. New York: Wiley.
38. Winokur, G., Clayton, P. J., & Reich, T. (1969). *Manic Depressive Illness*. St. Louis: Mosby.
39. Wurtman, R. (1982, April). Nutrients that modify brain function. *Scientific American*, pp. 50–59.
40. Wurtman, J. J., Wurtman, R., Growdon, J., et al. (1982). Carbohydrate craving in obese people: Suppression by treatments affecting serotonergic transmission. *International Journal of Eating Disorders, 1*, 2–15.

CHAPTER 4

1. Charney, D. S., Woods, S. W., Goodman, W. K., et al. (1986). The comparative efficacy of imipramine, alprazolam, and trazodone. *Journal of Clinical Psychiatry, 47*(12), 580–586.
2. Fisher, K. (1985, March). ECT: New studies on how, why, who. *APA Monitor*, pp. 18–19.
3. Fishman, S. M., & Sheehan, D. V. (1985, April). Anxiety and panic: Their cause and treatment. *Psychology Today*, pp. 26–32.
4. Jimerson, D. C. (1987). Role of dopamine mechanisms in the affective disorders. In H. Y. Meltzer (Ed.), *Psychopharmacology: The Third Generation of Progress* (pp. 505–511). New York: Raven Press.
5. Mishra, R., & Sulser, F. (1978). Role of serotonin reuptake inhibition in the development of subsensitivity of the norepinephrine (NE) receptor coupled adenylate system. *Communications in Psychopharmacology, 2*, 365–370.
6. Mishra, R., Janowsky, A., & Sulser, F. (1980). Action of mianserin and zimelidine on the norepinephrine receptor coupled adenylate cyclase system in brain: Subsensitivity without reduction in β-adrenergic receptor binding. *Neuropharmacology, 19*, 983–987.
7. National Institute of Mental Health. (1985). *Electroconvulsive Therapy: A Consensus Statement*. Bethesda, MD: U.S. Department of Health and Human Services.

8. Perse, T. (1988). Obsessive-compulsive disorder: A treatment review. *Journal of Clinical Psychiatry, 49*(2), 48–55.
9. Sackem, H. A. (1985, June). The case for ECT. *Psychology Today*, pp.37–40.
10. Smith, F. (1988, December 13). Electroshock: Controversial therapy is making a comeback. *San Jose Mercury News*, pp. 1C, 3C.
11. Snyder, S. H. (1980). *Biological Aspects of Mental Disorder*. New York: Oxford.

CHAPTER 5

1. Beck, A. T., Rush, A. J., Shaw, B., & Emery, G. (1979). *Cognitive Therapy of Depression: A Treatment Manual*. New York: Guilford Press.
2. Bergin, A., & Lambert, M. (1978). The evaluation of therapuetic outcomes. In S. Garfield & A. Bergin (Eds.), *Handbook of Psychotherapy and Behavior Change*. New York: Wiley.
3. DeAngelis, T. (1987, August). Short-term therapy is "magical" choice for many patients. *APA Monitor*.
4. Eysenck, H. J. (1952). The effects of psychotherapy: An evaluation. *Journal of Consulting Psychology, 16*, 319– 324.
5. Gallo, P. S. (1978). Meta-analysis—A mixed meta-phor? *American Psychologist, 33*, 515-517.
6. Haley, J. (1963). *Strategies of Psychotherapy*. New York: Grune & Stratton.
7. Howard, K. I., Kopta, S. M., Krause, M. S., & Orlinsky, D. E. (1986). The dose-effect in relationship in psychotherapy. *American Psychologist, 41*(2), 159–164.
8. Klerman, G. L., Weissman, M. M., Rounsaville, B. J., & Chevron, E. S. (1984). *Interpersonal Psychotherapy of Depression*. New York: Basic Books.
9. Meehl, P. E. (1955). Psychotherapy. *Annual Review of Psychology, 6*, 357–378.
10. Morrow-Bradley, C., & Elliot, R. (1986). Utilization of psychotherapy research by practicing psychotherapists. *American Psychologist, 41*(2), 188–197.
11. O'Connell, S. O. (1983). The placebo effect and psychotherapy. *Psychotherapy, Theory, Research, and Practice, 20*(3), 337–345.
12. Osler, W. (1906). *Aequanimitas*. New York: McGraw-Hill.
13. Perse, T. (1988). Obsessive-compulsive disorder: A treatment review. *Journal of Clinical Psychiatry, 49*(2), 48–55.
14. Raimy, B. (Ed.). (1950). *Training in Clinical Psychology*. New York: Prentice-Hall.
15. Shapiro, A. K., & Morris, L. A. (1978). Placebo effects in medicine, psycho-therapy, and psychanalysis. In S. L. Garfield & A. E. Bergin (Eds.), *Handbook of Psychotherapy and Behavior Change: An Empirical Analysis* (2nd ed., pp. 369–410). New York: Wiley.
16. Shapiro, D. A., & Shapiro, D. (1982). Meta-analysis of comparative therapy out-come studies: A replication and refinement. *Psychological Bulletin, 92*(3), 581-604.
17. Shapiro, S., Skinner, E. A., Kessler, L. G., et al. (1984). Utilization of health and mental health services. *Archives of General Psychiatry, 41*, 971–978.
18. Smith, M. L., & Glass, G. V. (1977). Meta-analysis of psychotherapy outcome studies. *American Psychologist, 32*, 752–760.
19. Stiles, W. B., Shapiro, D. A., & Elliot, R. (1986). "Are all psychotherapies equivilent?" *American Psychologist, 41*(2), 165–180.

20. Strupp, H. H., & Hadley, S. W. (1979). Specific vs. nonspecific factors in psychotherapy. *Archives of General Psychiatry, 36,* 1125–1138.
21. Taube, C. A., Burns, B. J., & Kessler, L. (1984). Patients of psychiatrists and psychologists in office-based pratice. *American Psychologist, 39*(12), 1435–1447.
22. Therapy effective as depression cure. (1986, May 14). *San Jose Mercury News,* pp. 1A, 14A.
23. Wiens, A. N., & Menustik, C. E. (1983, October). Treatment outcome and patient characteristics in an aversion therapy program for alcoholism. *American Psychologist,* pp. 1089–1121.

CHAPTER 6

1. Appenzeller, O., & Schade, D. R. (1979). Neurology of endurance training: 3. Sympathetic activity during a marathon race [Abstract]. *Neurology, 29,* 542.
2. Appenzeller, O., Standefer, J., Appenzeller, J., et al. (1980). Neurology of endurance training: Endorphins. *Neurology, 30,* 418–419.
3. Barchas, J., & Freedman, D. (1962). Brain amines: Response to physiological stress. *Biochemical Pharmocology, 12,* 1232–1235.
4. Berger, B. G., & Owen, D. R. (1983). Mood alteration with swimming—Swimmers really do "feel better." *Psychsomatic Medicine, 45*(5), 425–433.
5. Berk, L. S., Tan, S. A., Anderson, C. L., et al. (1981). Beta-endorphin response to exercise in athletes and nonathletes [abstract]. *Medicine and Science in Sports and Exercise, 13*(2), 134.
6. Bortz, W., II. (1982, April). The runner's high. *Runner's World,* pp. 58–88.
7. Brown, B. S., & Van Huss, W. D. (1973). Exercise and brain catecholamines. *Journal of Applied Physiology, 34,* 664– 669.
8. Brown, B. S., Payne, T., Kin, C., Moore, P., & Martin, W. (1979). Chronic response of rat brain norepinephrine and serotonin levels of endurance training. *Journal of Applied Physiology, 46,* 19–23.
9. Brown, R. S. (1987). Exercise as an adjunct to the treatment of mental disorders. In W. P. Morgan & S. E. Goldston (Eds.), *Exercise and Mental Health* (pp. 131–137). Washington, DC: Hemisphere.
10. Brown, R. S., Ramirez, D. E., & Taub, J. M. (1978, December). The prescription of exercise for depression. *The Physician and Sportsmedicine,* pp. 35–4511.
11. Carr, D. B., Bullen, B. A., Skrinar, G. S., Arnold, M. A., Rosenblatt, M., Beitins, I. Z., Martin, J. B., & MacArthur, J. W. (1981). Physical conditioning facilitates the exercise-induced secretion of beta-endorphins and betalipotropin in women. *New England Journal of Medicine, 305,* 560–562.
12. Christie, M. J., & Chesher, G. B. (1982). Physical dependence on physiologically released endogenous opiates. *Life Science, 30,* 1173–1177.
13. Clark, D. S., & Teasdale, J. D. (1982). Diurnal variation in clinical depression and accessibility of positive and negative experience. *Journal of Abnormal Psychologgy, 91,* 87–95.
14. Clark, M. S., Milberg, S., & Ross, J. (1983). Arousal cues arousal-related material in memory: Implications for understanding effects of mood on memory. *Journal of Verbal Learning and Verbal Behavior, 22,* 633–649.

15. Denton, L. (1987, November). Mood's role in memory still puzzling. *APA Monitor*.

16. Doctor, R., & Sharkey, B. J. (1971). Note on some physiological and subjective reactions to exercise and training. *Perception and Motor Skills, 32*, 233–237.

17. Doyne, E. J., Chambless, D. L., & Beutler, L. E. (1983). Aerobic exercise as a treatment for depression in women. *Behavior Therapy, 14*, 434–440.

18. Farrell, P. K., Gates, W. K., Maksud, M. G., et al. (1982). Increases in plama β-endorphin/β-lipotropin immunoreactivity after treadmill running in humans. *Journal of Applied Physiology, 52*, 1245–1249.

19. Farrell, P. K., Gates, W. K., and Morgan, W. P., et al. (1983). Plasma leucine enkephalin-like radioreceptor activity and tension-anxiety before and after competitive running. In H. G. Knuttgen, J. A. Vogel, & J. Poortmans (Eds.), *Biochemistry of Exercise*. Champaign, Ill: Human Kinetics.

20. Fawcett, J., Mass, J. W., & Dekirmenjiar, H. (1972). Depression and MHPG excretion. *Achives of General Psychiatry, 26*, 246–251.

21. Fremont, J., & Craighead, L. W. (1984). *Aerobic Exercise and Cognitive Therapy for Mild/Moderate Depression*. Presented at the Association for Advancement of Behavior Therapy, Philadelphia.

22. Garver, D. L., & Davis, J. M. (1979). Minireview: Biogenic amine hypotheses of affective disorders. *Life Sciences, 24*, 383–394. Pergamon Press.

23. Glowinski, J., & Axelrod, J. (1964). Inhibition of uptake of titrated noradrenaline in the intact rat brain by imipramine and structurally related compounds. *Nature, 204*, 1318–1319.

24. Glowinski, J., & Baldessarini, R. J. (1966). Metabolism of norepinephrine in the central nervous system. *Pharmocology Review, 18*, 1201–1238.

25. Graham-Smith, D. G., Green, A. R., & Costain, D. W. (1978). Mechanism of antidepressant action of electro-convulsive therapy. *Lancet, 1*, 254–256.

26. Greist, J. H., Klein, M. H., Eischens, R. R., & Faris, J. T. (1978, December). Running out of depression. *The Physician and Sportsmedicine*, pp.49–56.

27. Greist, J. H., Klein, M. H., Eischens, R. R., Faris, J. T., Gurman, A. S., & Morgan, W. P. (1979). Running as a treatment for depression. *Comprehensive Psychiatry, 20*, 41–54.

28. Haier, R. J., Quaid, B. A., & Mills, J. S. (1981). Naloxone alters pain perceptions after jogging [Letter]. *Psychiatric Research, 5*, 231–232.

29. Howley, E. T. (1981). The excretion of catecholamines as an index of exercise stress. In F. J. Nagel & H. J. Montoye (Eds.), *Exercise in Health and Disease*. Springfield, IL: Charles C Thomas.

30. Kavanagh, T., Shephard, R., & Tuck, J. (1975, July). Depression after myocardial infarction. *Canadian Medical Association Journal, 113*, 23–27.

31. Klein, M. K., Greist, J. H., Gurman, A. S., Neimeyer, R. A., Lesser, D.P., Bushnell, N. J., & Smith, R. E. (1985). A comparative outcome study of group psychotherapy vs. exercise treatments for depression. *International Journal of Mental Health, 13*(3–4), 148–177.

32. Lilliefors, J. (1978). *The Running Mind*. Mountain View, CA: World.

33. Lloyd, G. G., & Lishman, W. A. (1975). Effect of depression on speed of recall of pleasant and unpleasant experiences. *Psychological Medicine, 5*, 73–180.

34. Lobstein, D. D., Mosbacher, B. J., & Ismail, A. H. (1983). Depression as a powerful discriminator between physcially active and sedentary middle-aged men. *Journal of Psychosomatic Research, 27*(1), 69–76.

35. Markoff, R. A., Ryan, P., & Young, T. (1982). Endorphins and mood changes in long-distance running. *Medicine and Science in Sports and Exercise, 14,* 11–15.

36. Martinsen, E. W. (1987). Exercise and medication in the psychiatric patient. In W. P. Morgan & S. E. Goldston (Eds.), *Exercise and Mental Health* (pp. 85–95). Washington, DC: Hemisphere.

37. McCann, I. L., & Holmes, D. S. (1984). The influence of aerobic exercise on depression. *Journal of Personality and Social Psychology, 46*(5), 1142–1147.

38. Morgan, W. P. (1985). Affective beneficence of vigorous physical activity. *Medicine and Science in Sports and Exercise, 17*(1), 94–100.

39. Pert, C. B., & Bowie, D. L. (1979). Behavioral manipulation of rats cause alterations in opiate receptor occupancy. In E. Usdin, W. E. Bunney, & N. S. Kline (Eds.), *Endorphins and Mental Health* (pp. 93–104). New York: Oxford University Press.

40. Pierce, D., Kupprat, I., & Harry, D. (1976). Urinary epinephrine and norepinephrine levels in women athletes training and competition. *European Journal of Applied Physiology, 36,* 1–6.

41. Ransford, C. P. (1982). A role for amines in the antidepressant effect of exercise: A review. *Medicine and Science in Sports and Exercise, 14,* 1–10.

42. Reuter, M., Mutrie, N., & Harris, D. V. (1984). *Running as an Adjunct to Counseling in the Treatment of Depression.* Unpublished manuscript, The Pennsylvania State University.

43. Sachs, M. L. (1980). *On the Trail of the Runner's High: A Descriptive and Experimental Investigation of Characteristics of an Elusive Phenomenon.* Ph.D. thesis, Florida State University.

44. Sime, W. E. (1987). Exercise in the prevention and treatment of depression. In W. P. Morgan & S. E. Goldston (Eds.), *Exercise and Mental Health* (pp. 145–152). Washington, DC: Hemisphere.

45. Simmons, A. D., Epstein, L. H., McGowan, C. R., Kupfer, D. J., & Robertson, R. J. (1985). Exercise as a treatment for depression: An update. *Clinical Psychology Review, 5,* 553–568.

46. Teasdale, J. D., Taylor, R., & Fogarty, S. J. (1980). Effects of induced elation-depression on the accessibility of memories of happy and unhappy exerperiences. *Behavior Research and Therapy, 18,* 339–346.

47. Tharp, G. D., & Carson, W. H. (1975). Emotionality changes in rats following chronic exercise. *Medicine and Science in Sports and Exercise, 7,* 123–126.

48. Tooman, M. E. (1982). *The Effect of Running and Its Deprivation on Muscle Tension, Mood, and Anxiety.* Unpublished master's thesis, The Pennsylvania State University.

49. Valtonen, E. J. (1968). Immediate effect of short wave diathermy on the 5-hydroxytryptamine content of blood and brain in the rat. *American Journal of Physiological Medicine, 47,* 171–174.

50. Wardlaw, S. L., & Frantz, A. G. (1980). Effect of swimming stress on brain B-endorphin and ACTH [Abstract]. *Clinical Research, 28,* 482.

51. Weber, J. C., & Lee, R. A. (1968). Effects of differing prepuberty exercise programs on the emotionality of male albino rats. *Research Quarterly, 39,* 748–751.
52. Weiss, J. M. (1982). *A Model of Neurochemical Study of Depression.* Paper presented at the Annual Convention of the American Psychological Association, Washington, DC.
53. Zeiss, L. P., & Munoz, R. (1979). Nonspecific improvement effects in depression using interpersonal skills training, pleasant activities schedules, or cognitive training. *Journal of Consulting and Clinical Psychology, 47,* 427–439.

CHAPTER 7

1. Anderson, C. M., & Stewart, S. (1983). *Mastering Resistance: A Practical Guide to Family Therapy.* New York: Guilford Press.
2. Erickson, M. H. (1959). Further clinical techniques of hypnosis: Utilization techniques. *American Journal of Clinical Hypnosis, 1,* 3–21.
3. Fisch, R., Weakland, J. H., & Segal, L. (1983). *The Tactics of Change: Doing Therapy Briefly.* San Francisco: Jossey-Bass.
4. Foley, V. D. (1984). Family therapy. In R. J. Corsini (Ed.), *Current Psychotherapies* (3rd ed., pp. 447–490). Itasca, IL: Peacock.
5. Haley, J. (1963). *Strategies of Psychotherapy.* New York: Grune & Stratton.
6. Haley, J. (1973). *Uncommon therapy: The Psychiatric Techniques of Milton Erickson, M.D.* New York: Norton.
7. Haley, J. (1976). *Problem-Solving Therapy.* San Francisco: Jossey-Bass.
8. Kostrubala, T. (1976). *The Joy of Running.* New York: J. B. Lippincott.
9. Omer, H., & London, P. (1988, Summer). Metamorphosis in psychotherapy: End of the systems era. *Psychotherapy, 25*(2), 171–182.
10. Palazzoli, M., Boscolo, L., Cecchin, G., & Prata, G. (1978). *Paradox and Counterparadox.* New York: Jason Aronson.
11. Sime, W. E. (1987). Exercise in the prevention and treatment of depression. In W. P. Morgan & S. E. Goldston (Eds.), *Exercise and Mental Health* (pp. 145–152). Washington, DC: Hemisphere.
12. Watzlawick, P., Weakland, J. E., & Fisch, R. (1974). *Change: Principles of Problem Formation and Problem Resolution.* New York: Norton.

CHAPTER 8

1. Bahrke, M. S., & Morgan, W. P. (1978). Anxiety reduction following exercise and meditation. *Cognitive Therapy Research, 2,* 223–233.
2. Brown, R. S. (1987). Exercise as an adjunct to the treatment of mental disorders. In W. P. Morgan & S. E. Goldston (Eds.), *Exercise and Mental Health* (pp. 131–137). Washington, DC: Hemisphere.
3. Cannon, J. G., & Kluger, M. J. (1983). Endogenous pyrogen activity in human plasma after exercise. *Science, 220,* 617–619.

4. de Vries, H. A. (1981). Tranquilizer effect of exercise: A critical review. *The Physician and Sportsmedicine, 9*(11), 46–55.
5. Dishman, R. K. (1985). Medical psychology in exercise and sport. *Medical Clinics of North America, 69*(1), 123–143.
6. Fasting, K., & Grønningsæter, H. (1986). Unemployment, trait anxiety, and physical exercise. *Scandinavian Journal of Sports Science, 8*(3), 99–103.
7. Morgan, W. P.(1979, March). Anxiety reduction following acute physical activity. *Psychiatric Annals, 9*(3), 36–45.
8. Orwin, A. (1973). The running treatment: A preliminary communication on a new use for an old therapy (physical activity) in the agoraphobic syndrome. *British Journal of Psychiatry, 122,* 175–179.
9. Orwin, A. (1974). Treatment of a situational phobia—A case for running. *British Journal of Psychiatry, 125,* 95–98.
10. Spielberger, C. D., Gorsuch, R. L., & Lushene, R. (1970). *State-Trait Anxiety Inventory Manual.* Palo Alto, CA: Consulting Psychologists Press.

CHAPTER 9

1. Appenzeller, O., & Schade, D. R. (1979). Neurology of endurance training: 3. Sympathetic activity during a marathon race [Abstract]. *Neurology, 29,* 542.
2. Ben-Shlomo, L. S., & Short, M. A. (1983). The effects of physical exercise on self-attitudes. *Occupational Therapy in Mental Health, 3*(4), 11–28.
3. Berger, B. G., & Owen, D. R. (1983). Mood alteration with swimming— Swimmers really do "feel better." *Psychosomatic Medicine, 45*(5), 425–433.
4. Boyll, J. R. (1986). The effects of active exercise and passive electronic muscle stimulation on self-concept, anxiety, and depression. (Doctoral disseration, Northern Arizona University). *Dissertation Abstracts International, 47*(5-B), 2219.
5. Brown, R. D. (1986). *Effects of a Strength Training Program on Strength, Body Composition, and Self-Concept of Females.* Doctoral dissertation, Brigham Young University.
6. Brown, R. S., Ramirez, D. E., & Taub, J. M. (1978, December). The prescription of exercise for depression. *The Physician and Sportsmedicine,* pp. 35–45.
7. Brown, R. S. (1987). Exercise as an adjunct to the treatment of mental disorders. In W. P. Morgan & S. E. Goldston (Eds.), *Exercise and Mental Health* (pp. 131–137). Washington, DC: Hemisphere.
8. Clark, B. A., Wade, M. G., Massey, B. H., & Van Dyke, R. (1975). Response of institutionalized geriatric mental patients to a twelve-week program of regular physical exercise. *Journal of Gerontology, 30,* 565–573.
9. Collingwood, T. R. (1972). The effects of physical training upon behavior and self attitudes. *Journal of Clinical Psychology, 28,* 583–585.
10. Collingwood, T. R., & Willet, L. (1971). The effects of physical training upon self-concept and body attitude. *Journal of Clinical Psychology, 27,* 411–412.
11. Dodson, L. C., & Mullens, W. R. (1969). Some effects of jogging on psychiatric hospital patients. *American Corrective Therapy Journal, 23,* 130–134.

12. Duke, M., Johnson, T. C., & Nowicki, S., Jr. (1977). Effects of sports fitness camp experience on locus of control orientation in children, ages 6 to 14. *Research Quarterly, 48*, 280–283.
13. Folkins, C. H., & Sime, W. E. (1981). Physical fitness training and mental health. *American Psychologist, 36*(4), 373–389.
14. Frankel, A., & Murphy, J. (1974). Physical fitness and personality in alcoholism. *Quarterly Journal of Studies on Alcoholism, 35*, 1272–1278.
15. Fremont, J., & Craighead, L. W. (1984). *Aerobic Exercise and Cognitive Therapy for Mild/Moderate Depression*. Presented at the Association for Advancement of Behavior Therapy, Philadelphia, PA.
16. Gary, V., & Guthrie, D. (1972). The effect of jogging on physical fitness and self-concept in hospitalized alcoholics. *Quarterly Journal of Studies on Alcoholism, 33*, 1073–1078.
17. Harris, D. V. (1973). *Involvement in Sports: A Somatopsychic Rationale for Physical Activity*. Philadelphia: Lea & Febiger.
18. Heaps, R. A. (1978). Relating physical and psychological fitness: A psychological point of view. *Journal of Sports Medicine and Physical Fitness, 18*, 399–408.
19. Hopson, J. L. (1988, July/August). A pleasureable chemistry. *Psychology Today*, pp. 29–33.
20. King, T. (1987). *The Effects of Exercise on Self-Esteem: A Review*. Unpublished manuscript, San Jose State University, Psychology Department.
21. Kostrubala, T. (1976). *The Joy of Running*. New York: Lippincott.
22. Kramer, R., & Bauer, R. (1955). Behavioral effects of hydrogymnastics. *Journal of the Association of Physical and Mental Rehabilitation, 9*, 10–12.
23. Layman, E. M. (1974). Psychological effects of physical activity. In J. H. Wilmore (Ed.), *Exercise and Sports Sciences Reviews*. New York: Academic Press.
24. Leonardson, G. R. (1977, September/October). Self-esteem: An important correlate of physical fitness. *Journal of Physical Education, 16*.
25. Murphy, J. B., Bennett, R. N., Hagen, J. M., & Russell, M. W. (1972). Some suggestive data regarding the relationship of physical fitness to emotional difficulties. *Newsletter for Research in Psychology, 14*, 15–17.
26. Powell, R. R. (1974). Psychological effects of exercise therapy upon institutionalized geriatric mental patients. *Journal of Gerontology, 29*, 157–161.
27. Powers, K. R. (1984). The effects of physical challenge training on self-concept and locus of control in women. (Doctoral dissertation, University of Pittsburg). *Dissertation Abstracts International, 44*(8-A), 2364.
28. Shipman, W. M. (1984). Emotional and behavioral effects of long-distance running on children. In M. L. Sachs & G. W. Buffone (Eds.), *Running as Therapy: An Integrated Approach*. Lincoln: University of Nebraska Press.
29. Sinyor, Y., Brown, T., Rostant, L., & Seraganian, P. (1982). The role of a physical fitness program in the treatment of alcoholism. *Journal of Studies on Alcohol, 43*, 380–386.
30. Smith, W. C., & Figetakis, N. (1970). Some effects of isometric exercise on muscular strength, body-image perception, and psychiatric symptomatology in chronic schizophrenics. *American Corrective Therapy Journal, 24*, 100–104.

31. Stamford, B. A., Hambacher, W., & Fallica, A. (1974). Effects of daily physical exercise on the psychiatric state of institutionalized geriatric mental patients. *Research Quarterly, 45,* 34–41.
32. Study: Active brains stay sharper. (1984, November 27). *San Jose Mercury News.*
33. Telander, R. (1988, October 17). Sports behind the walls. *Sports Illustrated.*
34. Timmerman, J. (1954). Effectiveness of hydrogymnastic therapy in treating the acutely disturbed psychotic. *Journal of the Association of Physical and Mental Rehabilitation, 8,* 192–194.
35. Trujillo, C. M. (1983). The effect of weight training and running exercise intervention programs on self-esteem of college women. *International Journal of Sports Psychology, 14,* 162–173.
36. Wilfley, D., & Kunce, J. T. (1986). Differential physical and psychological effects of exercise. *Journal of Counseling Psychology, 33*(3), 337–342.

CHAPTER 10

1. Aloia, J. F., Cohn, S. H., Babu, T., *et al.* (1978). Skeletal mass and body composition in marathon runners. *Metabolism, 27,* 1793–1796.
2. Aloia, J. F., Cohn, S. H., Ostuni, J. A., *et al.* (1978) Prevention of involutional bone loss by exercise. *Annals of Internal Medicine, 89,* 356–358.
3. Bier, D. M., & Young, V. R. (1983). Exercise and blood pressure: Nutritional considerations. *Annals of Internal Medicine, 98* (Part 2), 864–869.
4. Birkhead, N. C., Blizzard, J. J., Issekutz, B., *et al.* (1966). *Effect of Exercise, Standing, Negative Trunk and Positive Skeletal Pressure on Bedrest Induced Orthostasis and Hypercalciuria,* Technical Report 66-6. Wright Patterson AFB, Ohio.
5. Blume, E. (1987, August). The great protein myth. *San Jose Mercury News,* pp. 1F, 3F.
6. Bortz, W. M., II. (1982). Disuse and aging. *Journal of the American Medical Association, 248*(10), 1203–1208.
7. Bortz, W. M., II. (1983, October). Running, diabetes, and age—A challenging combination. *Fifty-Plus Bulletin,* p. 4.
8. Cohen, J. L., & Segal, K. R. (1984). Left ventricular hypertrophy in athletes: An exercise-echocardiographic study. *Medicine and Science in Sports, 17*(6), 695–700.
9. Costill, D. L. (1978, July). Coffee makes longer easier. *Runner's World,* p. 52.
10. Costill, D. L. (1979). *A Scientific Approach to Distance Running.* Los Altos: Track & Field News.
11. Dalen, N., & Olsson, K. C. (1974). Bone mineral content and physical activity. *Acta Orthopedics Scandinavia, 45,* 170–174.
12. Dishman, R. K. (1985). Medical psychology in exercise and sport. *Medical Clinics of North America, 69*(1), 123–143.
13. Donahoe, C. P., Lin, D. H., Kirschenbaum, D. S., *et al.* (1984). Metabolic consequences of dieting and exercise in the treatment of obesity. *Journal of Consulting and Clinical Psychology, 52*(5), 827–836.
14. Epstein, L. H., Wing, R. R., Koeske, R., *et al.* (1985). A comparison of lifestyle exercise, aerobic exercise, and calisthenics on weight loss in obese children. *Behavior Therapy, 16,* 345–356.

15. Franklin, D. (1986, July 30). Calcium may not help against osteoporosis. *San Jose Mercury News*, p. 13A.
16. Gauthier, M. (1986). Can exercise reduce the risk of cancer? *The Physician and Sportsmedicine, 14*(10), 171–178.
17. Hart, T. (1985, May). Of hearts and minds. *The Runner*, pp. 72–75.
18. Hartung, H., & Foreyt, J. (1983). Effect of alcohol intake on high density lipoprotein cholesterol levels in runners and inactive men. *Journal of the American Medical Association, 249*(6), 747–750.
19. Haskell, W. L. (1987). Developing an activity plan for improving health. In W. P. Morgan & S. E. Goldston (Eds.), *Exercise and Mental Health*, (pp. 37–55). Washington, DC: Hemisphere.
20. Higdon, H. (1987, December). In with the good. *Runner's World*, pp. 50–54.
21. Howley, E. T., & Glover, E. G. (1974). The caloric costs of running and walking one mile for men and women. *Medicine and Science in Sports, 6*, 235–237.
22. Jeffery, D., & Katz, R. (1977). *Take It Off and Keep It Off: A Behavioral Program for Weight Loss and Healthy Living*. Englewood Cliffs, NJ: Prentice-Hall.
23. Kramsch, D. M., Aspen, A. J., Abramowitz, B. M., et al. (1981). Reduction of coronary artherosclerosis by moderate conditioning exercise in monkeys on an atherogenic diet. *New England Journal of Medicine, 305*(25), 1483–1498.
24. Krauss, R., Williams, P., Lindgren, F., & Wood, P. (1988). Coorinate changes in levels of human serum low and high density lipoprotein subclasses in healthy men. *Arteriosclerosis, 8*(2), 155–162.
25. Kolata, G. (1987). Metabolic catch-22 of exercise regimens. *Science, 236*, 146–147.
26. Lane, N. E., Bloch, D. A., Jones, H. H., et al. (1986). Long-distance running, bone density, and osteoarthritis. *Journal of the American Medical Association, 255*(9), 1147–1151.
27. Leary, W. E. (1989, January 13). Spinal osteoporosis is halted in breakthrough study says. *San Jose Mercury News*, pp. 1A, 13A.
28. McCunney, R. J. (1987). Fitness, heart disease, and high density lipoproteins: A look at the relationships. *The Physician and Sportsmedicine, 15*(2), 67–79.
29. McGuire, R. (1988, July 13). Cholesterol and blood pressure. *San Jose Mercury News*.
30. Minaire, P., Neunier, P. Edouard, C., et al. (1974). Quantitative histological data on disuse osteoporisis. *Calcification Disease Research, 17*, 57-73.
31. Morris, J. N., Kagan, A., Pattison, D. C., & Gardner, M. J. (1966). Incidence and prediction of ischaemic heartdisease in London busmen. *Lancet, 2*, 552–559.
32. Morris, J. N., Chave, S., Adam, C., et al. (1973). Vigorous exercise in leisure-time and the incidence of coronary heart-disease. *Lancet, 1*, 333–339.
33. Nadel, E. R. (1985). Physiological adaptations to aerobic training. *American Scientist, 73*, 334–343.
34. Obesity is a "killer" disease, health panel warns. (1985, January 1). *San Jose Mercury News*.
35. Pacy, P. J., Webster, J., & Garrow, J. S. (1986). Exercise and obesity. *Sports Medicine, 3*, 89–113.
36. Paffenbarger, R. S., Brand, R. J., Sholtz, R. I., et al. (1978). Energy expenditure, cigarette smoking, and blood pressure level as related to death from specific diseases. *American Journal of Epidemiology, 108*(1), 12–18.

37. Paffenbarger, R. S., Hyde, R. T., Wing, A. L., et al. (1986). Physical activity, all-cause mortality, and longevity of college alumni. *New England Journal of Medicine, 314,* 605– 613.

38. Raeburn, P. (1988, October 5). Intense exercise can be bad for women's bones. *San Jose Mercury News,* p. 2F.

39. Randall, F. (1982, July). Getting to the heart of the matter. *The Runner,* pp. 80–86.

40. Rogers-Gould, G. (1987, September 9). How exercise keeps cancer away. *San Jose Mercury News,* p. 2E.

41. Sidney, S., Friedman, G. D., & Hiatt, R. A. (1986). Serum cholesterol and large bowel cancer. *American Journal of Epidemiology, 124*(1), 33–38.

42. Smith, E. L. (1973). The effects of physical activity on bone in the aged. In R. B. Mazess (Ed.), *International Conference on Bone Mineral Measurement* (pp. 397–407). Washington, DC: DHEW Pub. No. (NIH) 75-683.

43. Smith, E. L., Reddan, W., & Smith, P. E. (1981). Physical activity and calcium modalities for bone mineral increase in aged women. *Medicine and Science in Sports and Exercise, 13,* 60–64.

44. Spitz, M. R. (1985). Cholesterol and cancer relationship. *The Cancer Bulletin of the University of Texas,* M. D. Anderson Hospital and Tumor Institute at Houston, *37*(May/ June), 114–116.

45. Study says calcium fails to stop bone loss by itself. (1987, January 13). *San Jose Mercury News,* p.3E.

46. Tipton, C. M., (1984). Exercise, training, and hypertension. In R. L. Terjung (Ed.), *Exercise and Sport Science Reviews, 12,* (pp. 245–306). New York: Macmillan.

47. Tran, Z. V., & Weltman, A. (1985). Differential effects of of exercise on serum lipid and lipoprotein levels seen with changes in body weight: A meta-analysis. *Journal of the American Medical Association, 254,* 2080–2086.

48. Watson, R. C. (1973). Bone growth and physical activity in young males. In R. B. Mazess (Ed.), *International Congress on Bone Mineral Measurement* (pp. 380–386). Washington DC: DHEW Pub. No. (NIH) 75-683. 380–386.

49. Whitaker, J. (1979, February). How much protein do runners need? *Runner's World,* pp. 64, 66.

50. Williams, J., Wagner, J., Wasnich, R., & Heilabrun, L. (1984). The effect of long-distance running upon appendicular bone mineral content. *Medicine and Science in Sports and Exercise, 16*(3), 223–227.

51. Williams, P., Wood, P., Haskell, W., & Vranizan, K. (1982). The effects of running mileage and duration on plasma lipoprotein levels. *Journal of the American Medical Association, 247*(19), 2674–2679.

52. Wood, P. D. (1979, June) Running away from heart disease: Becoming familar with your lipoproteins could save your life. *Runner's World,* pp. 78–81.

53. Wood, P. D. (1979, December) Does running help prevent heart attacks? *Runner's World,* pp. 85–91.

54. Wood, P. D. (1980, September) The eat-more, weigh-less diet. *Runner's World,* pp.42–44.

55. Wood, P. D. (1983). *California Diet and Exercise Program.* Mountain View, CA: Anderson World Books.

56. Wood, P. D., & Haskell, W. L. (1979). The effect of exercise on plasma high density lipoproteins. *Lipids*, *14*(4), 417–427.
57. Wood, P. D., Haskell, W. L., & Klein, H. (1976). The distribution of plasma lipids in middle aged male runners. *Metabolism*, *25*, 1249-1257.
58. Wood, P. D., Stefanick, M., Dreon, D., *et al.* (1988, November 3). Changes in plasma lipids and lipoproteins in overweight men during weight loss through dieting as compared with exercise. *New England Journal of Medicine*, *319*, 1173–1179.

CHAPTER 11

1. Baekeland, F. (1970). Exercise deprivation. *Archives of General Psychiatry*, *22*, 365–369.
2. Carmack, M. A., & Martens, R. (1979). Measuring commitment to running: A survey of runner's attitudes and mental states. *Journal of Sports Psychology*, *1*, 25–42.
3. Chang, J. L., Blumenthal, J. A., & O'Toole, L. C. (1984). Running and anorexia revisited: An empirical study of obligatory running and anorexia nervosa [Abstract]. *Medicine and Science in Sports and Exercise*, *16*, 172.
4. Collu, R., Ducharme, J. P., Barbeau, A., *et al.* (Eds.). (1982). *Brain Neurotransmitters and Hormones*. New York: Raven Press.
5. Cooper, K. H. (1985, August). Running without fear. *The Runner*, pp. 68–73.
6. Costar, E. D. (1983, November). Eating disorders: Gymnastics at risk. *International Gymnastics*, 58–59.
7. Dishman, R. K. (1985). Medical psychology in exercise and sport. *Medical Clinics of North America*, *69*(1), 123-143.
8. Enns, M, Hinz, K., Clark, J., *et al.* (1983). Body composition, body size estimation and attitudes towards eating in male college athletes. In *Abstracts of the Fourth International Congress on Obesity*.
9. Friedman, M., Manwaring, J., Rosenman, R., *et al.* (1973). Instantaneous and sudden deaths, clinical and pathological differentiation in coronary artery disease. *Journal of the American Medical Association*, *225*, 1319–1328.
10. Garner, D., & Garfinkel, P. E. (1980). Social-cultural factors in the development of anorexia nervosa. *Psychological Medicine*, *10*, 647–656.
11. Garver, D. L., & Davis, J. M. (1979). Minireview: Biogenic amine hyptheses of affective disorders. *Life Sciences*, *24*, 383–394. Pergamon Press.
12. Gibbons, L. W., Cooper, K. H., Meyer, B. M., *et al.* (1980). The acute cardiac risk of strenuous exercise. *Journal of the American Medical Association*, *244*(16), 1799–1801.
13. Glasser, W. (1976). *Positive Addiction*. New York: Harper & Row.
14. Koplan, J. P. (1979). Cardiovascular deaths while running. *Journal of the American Medical Association*, *242*(23), 2578–2579.
15. Lane, N. E., Bloch, D. A., Jones, H. H., *et al.* (1986). Long-distance running, bone density, and osteoarthritis. *Journal of the American Medical Association*, *255*(9), 1147–1151.

16. Morgan, W. P. (1979). Negative addiction in runners. *The Physician and Sports-medicine, 7*, 57–70.

17. Olsen, E. (1982, May). Fitness report from the morgue. *The Runner*, pp. 57–63.

18. Opie, L. H. (1975). Sudden death and sport. *Lancet, 1*, 263–266.

19. Panush, R. S., Schmidt, C., Caldwell, J. R., *et al.* (1986). Is running associated with degenerative joint disease? *Journal of the American Medical Association, 255*(9), 1152– 1154.

20. Pargman, D. (1971). Body build and dietary habits in college athletes. *Medicine and Science in Sports and Exercise, 3*, 140–142.

21. Perse, T. (1988). Obsessive-compulsive disorder: A treatment review. *Journal of Clinical Psychiatry, 49*(2), 48–55.

22. Ragosta, M., Crabtree, J., Sturner, W., *et al.* (1983). Death during recreational exercise in the State of Rhode Island. *Medicine and Science in Sports and Exercise, 16*(4), 339– 342.

23. Sheehan, G. (1985, January). The heart of the matter. *The Runner*, pp. 12–13.

24. Siscovick, D. S., Weiss, N. S., Hallstrom, A. P., *et al.* (1982). Physical activity and primary cardiac arrest. *Journal of the American Medical Association, 248*(23), 3113–3117.

25. Thaxton, L. (1982). Physiological and psychological effects of short-term exercise addiction on habitual runners. *Journal of Sports Psychology, 4*, 73–80.

26. Wheeler, G. D., Conger, P., Wall, S. R., *et al.* (1984). Male distance runners: Correlation of psychological testing, eating attitudes, body image estimation, and serum testosterone [Abstract]. *Medicine and Science in Sports and Exercise, 16*, 172.

27. Yates, R. J., ALechey, K., & Shisslak, C. (1983). Running—An analogue of anorexia? *New England Journal of Medicine, 308*, 251–255.

CHAPTER 12

1. American College of Sports Medicine: Position statement on the recommended quantity and quality of exercise for developing and maintaining fitness in healthy adults. (1979). *Medicine and Science in Sports and Exercise, 10*, 7–10.

2. American College of Sports Medicine: Position statement on proper and improper weight loss programs. (1983). *Medicine and Science in Sports and Exercise, 15*(1), ix–xiii.

3. Berger, B. (1987). Stress levels in swimmers. In W. P. Morgan & S. E. Goldston (Eds.), *Exercise and Mental Health*. Washington, DC: Hemisphere.

4. Morain, C. (1988, July 13). Stop and go. *San Jose Mercury News*, pp. 1D, 3D.

5. Pocari, J., McCarron, R., Kline, G., *et al.* (1987). Is fast walking an adequate aerobic training stimulus for 30- to 69-year-old men and women? (1987). *The Physician and Sportsmedicine, 15*(2), 119–129.

6. Sullivan, B. (1988, December 11). When picking a sport, Americans are all wet. *San Jose Mercury News*, p. 9L.

7. Zuckerman, M. (1979). *Sensation Seeking: Beyond the Optimal Level of Arousal*. Hillsdale, NJ: Erlbaum.

Index

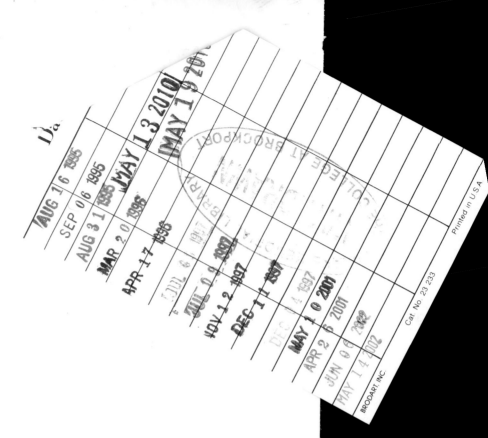